theclinics.com

CLINICS IN GERIATRIC MEDICINE

Alzheimer's Disease and Dementia

GUEST EDITOR
David S. Geldmacher, MD

February 2004 • Volume 20 • Number 1

SAUNDERS

An Imprint of Elsevier, Inc.
PHILADELPHIA LONDON TORONTO MONTREAL SYDNEY TOKYO

W.B. SAUNDERS COMPANY
A Division of Elsevier Inc.

The Curtis Center • Independence Square West • Philadelphia, PA 19106-3399

http://www.theclinics.com

CLINICS IN GERIATRIC MEDICINE **Volume 20, Number 1**
February 2004 **ISSN 0749-0690**
Editor: Elizabeth Bennett-Bailey

Clinics in Geriatric Medicine (ISSN 0749-0690) is published quarterly by W.B. Saunders Company. Corporate and editorial offices: The Curtis Center, Independence Square West, Philadelphia, PA 19106-3399. Accounting and circulation offices: 6277 Sea Harbor Drive, Orlando, FL 32887-4800. Periodicals postage paid at Orlando, FL 32862, and additional mailing offices. Subscription price is $156.00 per year (US individuals), $237.00 per year (US institutions), $196.00 per year (Canadian individuals), $292.00 per year (Canadian institutions), $202.00 per year (foreign individuals), and $292.00 per year (foreign institutions). Foreign air speed delivery is included in all *Clinics* subscription prices. All prices are subject to change without notice. POSTMASTER: Send address changes to *Clinics in Geriatric Medicine* W.B. Saunders Company, Periodicals Fulfillment, Orlando, FL 32887-4800. **Customer Service: 1-800-654-2452 (US). From outside of the US, call 1-407-345-4000. E-mail:hhspcs@harcourt.com.**

Clinics in Geriatric Medicine is covered in *Index Medicus, EMBASE/Excerpta Medica, Current Contents/Clinical Medicine (CC/CM), and the Cumulative Index to Nursing & Allied Health Literature.*

Printed in the United States of America.

GUEST EDITOR

DAVID S. GELDMACHER, MD, Associate Professor; and Director, Memory Disorders Program, Department of Neurology, University of Virginia Health System, Charlottesville, Virginia

CONTRIBUTORS

DAVID A. BENNETT, MD, Director, Rush Alzheimer's Disease Center; and Robert C. Borwell Professor, Department of Neurological Sciences, Rush Presbyterian–St. Luke's Medical Center, Chicago, Illinois

ELIZABETH A. CROOKS, RN, MSN, CCRN, CS, Doctoral Student, Frances Payne Bolton School of Nursing, Case Western Reserve University, Cleveland, Ohio

DAVID V. ESPINO, MD, Professor and Vice Chair for Community Geriatrics, Department of Family & Community Medicine, University of Texas Health Science Center, San Antonio, Texas

MARTIN R. FARLOW, MD, Professor, Department of Neurology, Indiana University School of Medicine, Indianapolis, Indiana

BARBARA FREUND, PhD, Assistant Professor of Medicine, Division of Geriatrics; and Director, Older Driver Research Program, The Glennan Center for Geriatrics and Gerontology, Eastern Virginia Medical School, Norfolk, Virginia

DAVID S. GELDMACHER, MD, Associate Professor and Director, Memory Disorders Program, Department of Neurology, University of Virginia Health System, Charlottesville, Virginia

STEFAN GRAVENSTEIN, MD, MPH, Professor of Medicine and Director, The Glennan Center for Geriatrics and Gerontology, Eastern Virginia Medical School, Norfolk, Virginia

KEVIN F. GRAY, MD, Associate Professor of Psychiatry and Instructor in Neurology, University of Texas Southwestern Medical Center; and Director, Geriatric Neuropsychiatry Clinic, Veterans Affairs North Texas Health Care System, Dallas, Texas

ANN MARIE HAKE, MD, Clinical Assistant Professor, Department of Neurology, Indiana University School of Medicine, Indianapolis, Indiana

SUZANNE HOLROYD, MD, Associate Professor, Director of Geriatric Psychiatry, Department of Psychiatric Medicine, University of Virginia, Charlottesville, Virginia

JENNIFER J. MANLY, PhD, Assistant Professor, Cognitive Neuroscience Division, Taub Institute for Research on Alzheimer's Disease & The Aging Brain, Columbia University Health Science Center, New York, New York

CAROL MANNING, PhD, Associate Professor of Neurology; and Director, Memory Disorders Clinic and Behavioral Neuropsychology Laboratory, Department of Neurology, University of Virginia Health System, Charlottesville, Virginia

DONNA MASTERMAN, MD, Associate Clinical Professor of Neurology, David Geffen School of Medicine at the University of California at Los Angeles, Los Angeles; and Associate Director, Early Development, Amgen, Inc., Thousand Oaks, California

CONTENTS

FORTHCOMING ISSUES

May 2004

Anti-Aging
Joseph H. Flaherty, MD, and
John E. Morley, MB, BCh, *Guest Editors*

August 2004

Incontinence
Mary M. Wilson, MD, *Guest Editor*

November 2004

Palliative Care I: Providing Care
Linda L. Emanuel, MD, PhD, *Guest Editor*

PREVIOUS ISSUES

November 2003

Geriatric Mental Health
George T. Grossberg, MD, *Guest Editor*

August 2003

Geriatric Sexuality
John E. Morley, MB, BCh, *Guest Editor*

May 2003

Osteoporosis
Ethel S. Siris, MD, *Guest Editor*

ELSEVIER
SAUNDERS

CLINICS IN
GERIATRIC
MEDICINE

Clin Geriatr Med 20 (2004) xi–xii

Preface

Alzheimer's disease and dementia

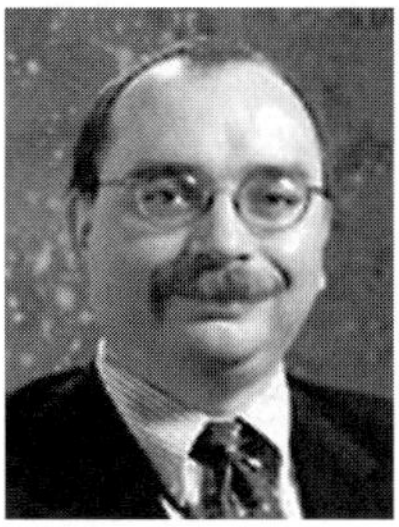

David S. Geldmacher, MD
Guest Editor

Is there really a need for another Alzheimer's disease update? A substantial amount of effort and resources go into putting together a focused issue of the *Clinics in Geriatric Medicine*. It should be clear from the publisher's and authors' commitment to this process, as well as my own perspective as Guest Editor, that—despite past updates—there remains a significant unmet need for knowledge about Alzheimer's disease (AD).

The explosion of information about AD continues unabated. The available material constitutes more than any person could reasonably synthesize from the primary literature. For example, in the interval from the publication of the last issue of the *Clinics in Geriatric Medicine* focusing on dementia, in 2001, through the development of this one for 2004, Medline lists over 6400 articles with "Alzheimer's disease" as key words. To complicate matters, the pace of the knowledge explosion is increasing. Looking only as far back as 5 and 10 years ago, Medline listed 6011 AD articles from 1996 to 1998 and "just" 3862 from 1991 to 1993.

Besides the sheer amount of information available, there have been other changes in the approach to AD in the last several years. The concept of mild cognitive impairment as a common prodromal state for dementia has risen in prominence. Evidence-based practice parameters for diagnosis and management of dementia have been updated or developed. New constructs for understanding the clinical and molecular biological expressions of fronto-temporal dementia and the tau-opathies have emerged. Longer-term studies of cholinesterase inhibitor drugs using outcomes more clinically relevant than simple cognitive test scores

0749-0690/04/$ – see front matter
doi:10.1016/j.cger.2003.11.005

have been reported. The hope for an "Alzheimer's vaccine" has blossomed and faded, perhaps soon to surface once again, re-energized. Past and foregone conclusions about estrogen and anti-inflammatory drugs have been challenged by new clinical trials and evidence-based critiques. Further revisions of assumptions and dogma are nearly guaranteed over the next several years as new therapeutic models further refine our understanding of the basic pathophysiologic processes associated with AD.

This issue tackles the great complexity of the field, distilling it to a level of practical use for the clinician caring for older adults at risk for, and with, dementing illness. The first articles focus on identifying and classifying cognitive impairments that may or may not represent incipient dementia. Recent viewpoints on syndromic, neuropsychological, and imaging approaches to dementia diagnosis follow. Management is addressed from the perspectives of cholinesterase inhibitors and handling difficult behaviors, to effective use of multidisciplinary resources. Special considerations for nursing home populations and cultural inclusiveness are incorporated. The issue concludes with a brief look to the short-term future of therapeutics for AD.

While much remains to be learned about AD, much can be done with what we know already. It is my hope that this issue will facilitate improved understanding of AD and allow implementation of better care of people and families affected by dementia today.

David S. Geldmacher, MD
Department of Neurology
University of Virginia Health System
P.O. Box 800394
Charlottesville, VA 22908, USA
E-mail address: dsg8n@virginia.edu

ELSEVIER
SAUNDERS

Clin Geriatr Med 20 (2004) 1–14

CLINICS IN
GERIATRIC
MEDICINE

Recognizing and evaluating potential dementia in office settings

Barbara Freund, PhD[a,b,*], Stefan Gravenstein, MD, MPH[c]

[a]*Division of Geriatrics, Eastern Virginia Medical School, 825 Fairfax Avenue, Suite 202, Norfolk, VA 23507, USA*

[b]*Older Driver Research Program, The Glennan Center for Geriatrics and Gerontology, Eastern Virginia Medical School, 825 Fairfax Avenue, Suite 202, Norfolk, VA 23507, USA*

[c]*The Glennan Center for Geriatrics and Gerontology, Eastern Virginia Medical School, 825 Fairfax Avenue, Suite 202, Norfolk, VA 23507, USA*

Cognitive impairment, the dementia prequel, and dementia itself are surprisingly prevalent among older, apparently healthy individuals. Cognitive impairment and dementia can each be detected in 10% of apparently healthy individuals over the age of 65 in an academic practice [1]. Dementia affects up to one third of people aged over 65 years but is overlooked in 25% to 90% [2–5]. Alzheimer's disease (AD) is the most common of the many dementias encountered in primary practice. In 2000, AD was estimated to afflict 4.5 million persons in the United States, a number expected to grow by 25% over the next 20 years, tripling to 13 million by 2050.

With the aging of the population, and the consequent growing prevalence of dementing illness in later life, primary care physicians will increasingly encounter a range of cognitive impairment in their patients. The generalist will need to incorporate a screening technique that is time- and cost-effective, and identifies those with a high likelihood of dementia for whom a full diagnostic work-up will be most appropriate to address and manage this incipient frailty.

Elements of the geriatric assessment for cognitive impairment

There are two specific challenges to the primary care physician in the context of dementia screening. First, how can the screening activity be fit into the framework of a routine office visit, both in the sense of best practice and economics of the primary care setting, and second, how can the screening activity direct the work-up for referral or additional testing before referral occurs? For the first

* Corresponding author. 825 Fairfax Avenue, Suite 202, Norfolk, VA 23507.
E-mail address: freundbm@evms.edu (B. Freund).

0749-0690/04/$ – see front matter
doi:10.1016/j.cger.2003.10.003

issue, fitting into the routine office visit, the screening activity must be both reliable and time efficient. For the second, the screening must be able to measure several aspects of cognition (eg, attention, memory, executive function), so that deficiencies in one or more areas would direct the follow-up.

Clinical assessment

Overview

Typically, the clinical assessment follows a patient or family report of memory problems. However, it is our contention that older primary care patients should be *routinely* screened for potential dementia. Even in the absence of apparent cognitive dysfunction, the older adult deserves a regular screening to detect cognitive impairment, and the interval between such assessments has been recommended to be as frequent as annually by some experts. To be practical, the screening activity needs to be targeted, efficient, and interpreted in the context of other contributing factors.

In a geriatrician's office, screening is often more detailed, and the patient is queried through a variety of means about abilities in activities of daily living, memory, behavior, chronology of symptoms, and any deviation from the usual level of performance. Additional components of the geriatric assessment include evaluations of balance and gait, social support, safety assessment, and advance directives. Although this is more comprehensive than most generalists are able to routinely incorporate in their clinical practices, elements can be culled for use in the generalist's office and be self-administered. The patient undergoes a brief clinical test of cognitive function followed by a general medical evaluation, directed at discovering systemic problems associated with confusion or delirium. Review of medications focuses particularly on drug interactions from polypharmacy and potential drug toxicities. The physician should perform a neurologic examination for detection of localizing signs and deep cortical involvement. When possible, the patient's family should be interviewed about activities of daily living, memory, behavior, chronology of symptoms, and any deviation from the patient's norm, and concordance with the patient report should be noted.

Initial recognition (screening)

Dementia screening is an activity that can be thought of similarly to screening for cardiac disease. In other words, the generalist can do for brain prevention the same as for cardioprevention. This sentiment as an approach to screening is gaining relevance as new prevention and treatment options become available. Unfortunately, the most widely used tools that are efficient lack a combination of high specificity and sensitivity. For this reason, the use of a single screening test will be impractical for the generalist as a comprehensive screening tool. The approach needs to consolidate and integrate screening, historical, and clinical

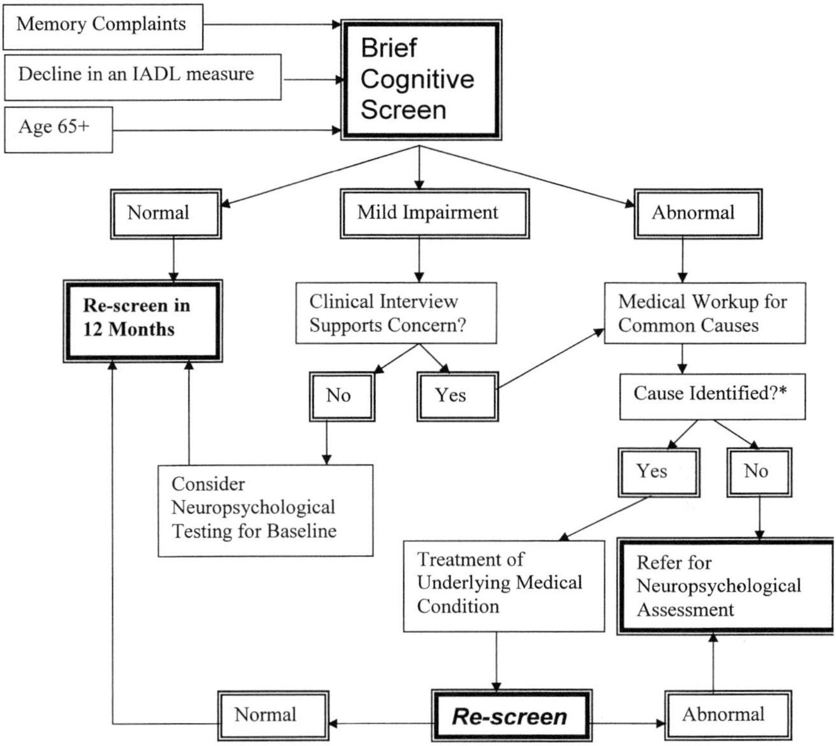

Fig. 1. Decision matrix for cognition screening.

information to adequately detect at-risk and demented subjects and to properly triage them through the decision matrix of whether to work-up in the office setting or refer (Fig. 1). A variety of screening tools are available for download at no charge at http://www.merckaging.com.

History

Common complaints that a general practitioner hears include memory lapses (early on in dementias, these are often nouns or names of people the patients should know), missed appointments, visual complaints discordant from ophthalmologic exam, hearing acuity problems, marital or family discord, new or expensive purchases, spousal/caregiver response to questions, history of falls, and incontinence. The history is essential to narrow the differential diagnosis by gathering clues from symptom duration and presentation.

Risk factors for cognitive impairment

Risk factors for dementia fall into three categories: aging, genes, and environment. These include such factors as advancing age, head trauma leading to loss of consciousness, vascular disorders (hypertension, cholesterol), alcohol abuse, diabetes, metabolic disorders, depression, encephalitis, meningitis, tuberculosis, syphilis, HIV, psychiatric hospitalization, postoperative delirium, stroke, heart disease, and certain malignancies. Family history of dementia, Parkinson's disease, psychiatric disease or hospitalization, cardiovascular disease, and stroke are also significant risk factors. For AD specifically, the primary risk factor is advancing age. Environmental factors related to AD include head injury and low-level education. Dementia, even subclinical dementia, is predisposed to delirium and transient delirium causes dementia if it is severe enough and long enough in duration (due to hypoxia and hypoglycemia, for example). However, the presence or absence of risk factors should not drive screening; it should be performed regardless because of the prevalence of significant subclinical impairment.

Cognition screening

The approach to "case detection" requires the implementation of a screening tool that can detect mild impairment. Two kinds of approaches may be appropriate depending on the resource availability. One could use an assessment tool that is completed by the patient or caregiver in the office; another approach could use an allied health professional to perform the screening event. Several tools have been validated for the office setting and are limited primarily by their relative sensitivity and specificity, and the usefulness of the data derived in sharing the information with other practitioners. Depending on the office setting, differing tools might be considered appropriate (Table 1).

The Mini-Mental State Exam (MMSE) is a well-known screen for cognitive impairment, particularly in the elderly. It is useful to document intellectual changes over time and is often used to assess the effects of cognition-enhancing therapies. It is relatively brief and easily scored. It is composed of items assessing orientation to time and place, attention and concentration, immediate

Table 1
Assessment tools for cognitive impairment

Tool/Setting	Solo practice	Nursing home	Geriatric team member	Neurologist, psychiatrist, psychologist	Time to administer (minutes)
MMSE	X	X	X	X	5–15
Clock Drawing	X		X		< 5
Geriatric Depression Scale	X		X	X	5–10
Trails A and B			X		5–10
Dementia Rating Scale			X		30–45
WMS/WAIS				X	>90
Caregiver stress			X		Variable
IADL, ADL	X	X	X		Variable
Safety	X		X		Variable

and delayed recall, language, and constructional ability. It is often used in primary care settings, although a common complaint is that it consumes too much of the already limited time the physician has with the patient.

The Clock Drawing Test (CDT) is a well-known, easily administered tool and is a useful measure of cognitive function [6–9]. The CDT relies on visuospatial, constructional and higher order cognitive abilities. Investigators using the CDT as a screen for dementia have developed several scoring scales. The CDT has been shown to correlate with executive control functions (the cognitive process necessary to plan and carry out goal-directed behaviors) [10], impairments of which are associated with functional disability and AD. It correlates well with disease progression [11] and is useful in the detection of very mild dementia [10]. It has also been shown to correlate moderately with driving performance [12], one of the higher level instrumental activities of daily living (IADL) functions and certainly one that is most challenging for physicians to assess. Subjects are instructed to draw a clock (free-hand is preferred to a predrawn circle), put all the numbers in, and set the time. There are different time-setting options depending upon which scoring method is used, although the time of 10 minutes past 11 o'clock is reported to be the most sensitive for detecting neurocognitive dysfunction [13].

The Geriatric Depression Scale (GDS) is a screening instrument to measure depression in the elderly (also referred to as the Mood Assessment Scale). The GDS is designed for self-administration. The subject is requested to complete a questionnaire referring to mood changes and to answer yes or no to descriptions of present feelings. The GDS takes approximately 5 to 10 minutes to complete. Cut-off points for the range of level of depression (normal through severely depressive) are recommended; however, it should be noted that this, along with the other tests described, is a screening rather than diagnostic test. Additional depression screening tools and diagnostic algorithms can be found at http://www.merckaging.com.

Trail Making Tests are tests of speed for attention, sequencing, mental flexibility, visual search, and motor function. The subject is required to connect 25 encircled numbers by pencil line (Part A) and 25 alternating encircled numbers and letters (Part B) in correct order. Administration takes approximately 5 to10 minutes. Tests are scored as the time in seconds required for each part. Limitations of these screening tools are presented in Table 2.

Other tests of cognitive function are too time intensive to be considered for use by the generalist. These tap into a variety of cognitive domains and would be administered in the referral setting. Examples include the Wechsler Memory Scale (WMS), the Wechsler Adult Intelligence Scale (WAIS), and the Blessed Test. For more information on these and other neuropsychologic testing instruments see elsewhere in this issue.

Positive screening for cognitive impairment does not necessarily mean a patient has dementia. It should trigger a comprehensive examination and referral as dictated by findings and practitioner experience. In addition to the routine physical examination, a detailed neurologic examination, neuropsychologic as-

Table 2
Characteristics of common cognition screening tools

Screening tool	Strengths	Weaknesses	Sensitivity	Specificity
MMSE	Well-known	Biased toward verbal items; inadequate measure of visuospatial ability, constructional praxis, ability to solve abstract problems or attend to relevant input; does not discriminate dementias	93% for scores $\geq$ 24 in subjects > 80 years; 100% for scores > 24 in subjects 65–69 years old; Decreases for scores < 24 [14]	42% for scores $\geq$ 24 in subjects > 80 years; 64% for scores > 24 in subjects 65–69 years old; Increases for scores < 24 [14]
CDT	Simple; tests multiple cognitive domains	May not discriminate dementias	91% [15]	95% [15]
Trails A	Tests rapid visual search	Does not discriminate dementias [16]	69% [16]	90% [16]
Trails B	Tests rapid visual search and set-shifting	More sensitive than Part A	87% [17]	88% [17]
GDS	Developed specifically for elderly; yes/no format lessens cognitive demands	Loses some validity in severe dementia	80% with cut-off of > 13 [18]	100% with cut-off of > 13 [18]

sessment, laboratory testing, and imaging are usually indicated. For many generalists, referral to a geriatrician, neurologist, psychiatrist, or psychologist for diagnosis and treatment recommendations, or to provide follow-along care occurs at this point because of constraints in time and skills.

Basic and instrumental activities of daily living

More than three decades ago, the World Health Organization recognized that "health in the elderly is best measured in terms of function [19]." Independent living represents the highest level of functional ability in older adults and can be compromised by a variety of factors. Because independent living requires the accomplishment of instrumental activities, conditions, such as dementia, that affect the ability to carry out the requisite tasks can contribute to functional decline. In fact, the severity of disease progression in dementia can be demonstrated by performance decline on IADL and ADL tasks. IADL performance decline has been associated with 1-year risk of incident dementia and is closely correlated with MMSE score [20]. The usual progression of decline is from higher level intellectual activities, such as money management, shopping, cooking, reading and driving, to lower level activities such as those addressing personal hygiene.

Functional status is reflected by performance on basic activities of daily living (self-care tasks such as bathing, grooming, and toileting) as well as instrumental activities of daily living (cognitively more complex activities such as driving and meal preparation that contribute to independent living). There are a number of validated scales for estimating functional ability [21–25]. The clinician may also ask the patient to describe a typical day and derive similar information. This can be followed by a request to describe how they like to spend leisure time, which requires recall of categories of activities and abstract thinking, cognitive abilities that decline early in AD. In the context of the cognitively impaired patient, corroborating the report with their caregiver or others in the position to know is important as such patients typically incorrectly report their participation in their IADLs and ADLs [26]. In our driving evaluation clinic, for example, the patients all indicate that they are excellent drivers.

Distinguishing the three Ds

An important consideration when the screening for cognitive impairment is positive is whether the impairment is associated with depression or delirium rather than dementia. Table 3 provides symptom distinctions between common cognition-impairing conditions. Depression may be the underlying or a significantly contributing cause of impairment, or it can accompany dementia as a direct result of neurologic damage. Delirium is characterized by sudden onset, altered consciousness, attention and concentration deficits out of proportion to other deficits, hallucinations, and intervals of lucidity. Delirium can be determined by using the Confusion Assessment Method (CAM) [27]. Almost always metabolic

Table 3
Distinctions between common causes of cognitive impairment[a]

	Mild cognitive impairment	Depression	Delirium	Dementia
Confusion	Absent	Absent	Present	
Attention	Good	Variable	Reduced	Good
Effort on tasks	Good	Reduced	Variable	Good
Consciousness	Clear	Clear, slowed	Clouded	Clear
Onset	Insidious	Recognized	Acute	Insidious
Duration	Months-years	Weeks-months	Acute	Months-years

[a] Focal neurologic causes present in < 10% delirium, metabolic encephalopathy.

in origin, delirium is commonly caused by medications, electrolyte imbalance, infection, and cerebral hypoperfusion. Delirium is often a complication of dementia, which further complicates distinguishing between the disorders.

Physical examination

Physical examination is directed toward the discovery and differentiation of conditions causing cognitive impairment, especially depression, delirium, and dementia (Table 4). The history will have substantially narrowed the differential diagnosis, as the chronicity and presentation provide useful clues. Focusing on metabolic (endocrine, toxic, medications, infectious, malignancy), vascular (connective tissue disease, stroke, peripheral vascular disease), and traumatic etiologies allows both a comprehensive and targeted approach. In addition, the generalist should observe the older patient's level of alertness, appearance, emotional state, and behavior, both mental and physical, as these will provide additional information about the patient's mental status and contribute to the differential diagnosis [28].

Patient safety

Patients with cognitive impairment are at risk for injury both inside and outside of their homes. The likelihood of risk is related to the severity of the impairment interfering with memory or appropriate judgment and decision-making. Inside the home, fire can result from forgotten pots left on the stove or careless smoking (lit cigarettes/cigars left in ashtrays, falling asleep while smoking). Additionally, the patient with impairment may not remember to call 911 for emergency assistance. Outside the home, patients can be injured if they wander and get lost and ask for help from strangers, or they can be involved in automobile accidents. For example, patients with dementia may not possess the insight to recognize declines in the ability to drive safely and may continue driving in the presence of moderate and even severe cognitive impairment [29]. Even patients with mild impairment may be experiencing declines in some aspects of driving that, while not significant enough to rescind driving privileges,

Table 4
Conditions associated with depression, delirium, and dementia

Condition	Examples of causes	Helpful physical findings	Special diagnostic studies
Depression	Hypothyroidism	Thickened hair, hung-up reflexes	TSH
	Prednisone, Cushing's disease	Osteoporosis, Dowager's hump, fractures	
Delirium	Hypermagnesemia	Drowsiness, diminished responsiveness, depressed or absent tendon reflexes, hypotension, respiratory depression, weakness	Magnesium
	Hypercalcemia	Band keratitis, hypotonia, weakness, fractures	Calcium
	Hypoglycemia	Polyuria, polyphagia, polydipsia, weakness, anorexia, nausea, disorientation	Glucose
	Hyperthyroidism, tranquilizers, narcotic, anticonvulsants, antineoplastic drugs, antipsychotic, etc.	Pupillary constriction, lethargy, increased tone, for example	TSH Tox screen
	Infection	Varies, depending on infectious agent and site of infection	RPR, HIV, TORCH, MRI
	Heavy metal	Varies, depending on metal	Mercury, lead, aluminum
Dementia	Alzheimer's disease,	No motor, focal findings	
	frontotemporal dementia, Pick's dementia,	Disinhibition, poor behavior control, cursing	
	Lewy body dementia	Parkinson-like motor findings, hallucinations	
	Multi-infarct dementia	Focal exam findings, atrial fibrillation, presence of bruits	Head CT or MRI
	Normal pressure hydrocephalus	Ataxia, incontinence	MRI, LP
	Vasculitis	Focal exam findings	ESR, ANA, LP, MRI
	Pernicious anemia	Proprioceptive loss	Methylmalonic acid, B12,
	Parkinson's disease	Cogwheeling, pill-rolling tremor, titubation, shuffling gait, retropulsion	
	Huntington's chorea	Choreoform movement	
	Subdural hematoma	Dysphasia	Head CT
	Syphilis	Cranial nerve palsies, stroke, ataxia, deep sensory loss	RPR, FTA-ABS, MRI
	Wernicke's encephalopathy	Confabulation, ophthalmoplegia -both lateral recti involved, sluggish pupils, truncal ataxia	Thiamine level

may require intervention in terms of driving restriction (short distances, daytime driving only, aided by co-pilot). Other safety issues are listed in Table 5.

Medications

Drugs, both therapeutic and toxic chemicals, are the most common reversible cause of cognitive impairment in older adults. This is due to the increased number of medications prescribed for the increased co-morbid conditions associated with aging as well as an enhanced sensitivity of the older brain to central nervous system effects of many medications, heavy metals, pesticides, and solvents. Table 6 provides a list of some of the more commonly prescribed drugs that affect cognition. Periodic evaluation of the patient's medications and modifications to optimize the simplest regimen that controls symptoms and disorders will result in risk reduction in terms of adverse events. A home evaluation by an allied

Table 5
Safety issues

Issue	Examples		
Driving	Going too fast or slow	Relies on passenger for instructions	Failure to observe traffic signs
	Frequent lane changes	Caused or involved in accident	Getting lost, especially in familiar areas
	Frequently replacing damaged or missing hubcaps		
Fires	Stove burners/oven left on	Burned pots/food	Careless smoking
	Inability to call for help in or exit in a fire		
Medications	Forgets medications	Hoards or hides medications	Takes wrong doses
	Takes someone else's medication	Alcohol abuse	
Wandering	Gets lost	Locks self outside the home	Stops strangers to take them home
	Improper clothing for weather		
Accidents	Falling	Injury using power equipment (saws, tools, guns, etc)	Poisoning (paints, solvents, insecticides, bleaches)
	Scalding while showering/bathing	Altering home temperature (turning off furnace)	
Food	Spoiled food	Forgetting to eat	Eating too much (not recalling they have already eaten)
Elder abuse	Accepting sales calls	Multiple duplicate subscriptions	Buying unnecessary items

Table 6
Examples of medications that adversely affect cognition

Classification	Example	Other confounding neurologic effects
Benzodiazepines	Diazepam, alprazolam	Sedation, daytime drowsiness
Neuroleptics	Clozapine, haloperidol, risperidone	Drowsiness, sedation, pseudoparkinsonism
Tricyclic-antidepressants	Amitriptyline, doxepin, desipramine, imipramine	Delusions, disorientation, insomnia, drowsiness
Antihistamines	Promethazine, diphenhydramine,	Drowsiness
Anti-Parkinsonian agents	Amantidine, levodopa, selegiline	Disorientation, confusion, hallucinations, depression
Antispasmodics	Metaclopromide, oxybutinin	Drowsiness, confusion, or excitement
Antiarrhythmics	Phenytoin, amiodarone, disopyramide	Tremor, light-headedness

health professional may be appropriate to evaluate medications sequestered over the years in the kitchen and bath cabinets.

Laboratory investigation

Clues on laboratory study of cognitive impairment include evidence for malnutrition, anemia, vitamin deficiency, renal and liver disease, infection, thyroid disorder, syphilis, and HIV. Specific tests to consider are presented in Table 7. In

Table 7
Laboratory studies

Laboratory test	Diagnosis	Comments
RPR[a]	Syphillis	If positive, consider FTA, HIV, head imaging
CMP[a]	Metabolic dysfunction	
CBC[a]	Anemia, malignancy, metabolic disease	
TSH[a]	Thyroid dysfunction	
B12[a], MMA	Vitamin B12 deficiency	
ESR	Vasculitis, connective tissue, and inflammatory disease	If abnormal consider ANA
Lipid panel/cascade[a]	Vascular risk factors	
Heavy metals	Heavy metal poisoning	If positive look for environmental causes
LP	Meningitis, Whipple's disease, MS, encephalitis, carinomatosis	
Folate	Folate deficiency	
UA	Urinary tract infection, metabolic dysfunction	
Drug screen	Drug toxicity, alcohol	
HIV	AIDS	Consider RPR, head imaging
EKG[a]	Cardiovascular disease, atrial fibrillation	
CT or MRI[a]	Mass, stroke, ischemic disease	

[a] Appropriate for a generalist to order in a routine dementia evaluation.

addition to the routine testing suggested, other tests can be ordered as indicated by the patients' clinical picture or as determined by the consultant.

Referrals

In the primary care office, detection of cognitive impairment should lead to a screening physical examination and laboratory testing to exclude common reversible causes of dementia. If the careful examination is nonfocal, laboratory testing normal, and history suggests a slowly progressive process over more than a year, the patient most likely has AD. Additional clinical findings can prompt additional testing or referral, as suggested in Table 4 or by the algorithm in Fig. 1. Any discomfort with the clinical exam or the diagnostic process or additional findings can prompt a referral to a clinician skilled in assessment and management of the patient with cognitive impairment. It is helpful to the consultant to receive the baseline information, including history, physical findings, and laboratory test results in forming an opinion on the first visit and being more selective on additional laboratory testing. Additional issues that the consultant may not address include those around safety concerns related to the cognitive impairment (see Table 5). Referral to a neuropsychologist is also appropriate, especially in mildly cognitively impaired individuals to establish a baseline level of dysfunction, support categorization into the type of dementia, and provide data for prognostication. Also, before referral, if medications or conditions, such as bladder infection or hypothyroidism, are identified that might interfere with cognition, they should be treated. The referral, barring crisis in patient behavior or other medical conditions, should be initiated when all test results are available. However, patients with immediate safety risks require immediate intervention addressing those risks.

Treatment options

If the comfort level is high, treatment with a dementia drug can be initiated, such as donepezil, tacrine, rivastigmine, galantamine, or memantine when available (see elsewhere in this issue for discussion of the decision matrix for treatment and benefit for non-AD dementia). Treatment, aside from anticholinesterase and glutamate therapy, for underlying causes such as depression, B12 deficiency, or hypothyroidis is also appropriate to initiate.

Summary

Cognitive impairment occurs along a continuum from mild to severe. Reports in the literature demonstrate that cognitive impairment across the continuum is largely unrecognized. In their review of studies comparing detection of dementia by standard diagnostic tests with documentation of dementia or cognitive impairment in the medical record, Boustani et al [30] found that 3.2% to 12% of patients 65 and older met criteria for dementia without documentation or physician knowledge of dementia. Further, they found that patients without a diagnosis of dementia represented 50% to 66% of all cases of dementia in the sample studies, and most of these were of mild to moderate severity. Cognitive impairment, if not frank dementia, often remains unrecognized until the cognitive symptoms have become severe. Impairments may be undiagnosed as many patients don't appear inappropriate in the context of a brief office visit. The challenge is to recognize impairment so that the increasingly available interventions can be provided early in the course of the illness, much the way cardiac and other symptoms in patients are now recognized early, or even before, frank symptoms have developed.

References

[1] Sager MA. Alzheimer's disease: research update. Keynote address. Annual Education Conference, Alzheimer's Association, Southeastern Virginia Chapter. June 5, 2003.

[2] Valcour VG, Masaki KH, Curb JD, Blanchette PL. The detection of dementia in the primary care setting. Arch Intern Med 2000;160:2964–8.

[3] Finkel SI. Cognitive screening in the primary care setting: the role of physicians at first point of entry. Geriatrics 2003;58(6):43–4.

[4] Ross GW, Abbott RD, Petrovitch H, et al. Frequency and characteristics of silent dementia among elderly Japanese-American men. The Honolulu-Asia Aging Study. JAMA 1997;277: 800–5.

[5] Callahan CM, Hendrie HC, Tierney WM. Documentation and evaluation of cognitive impairment in elderly primary care patients. Ann Intern Med 1995;122:422–9.

[6] Wolf-Klein GP, Silverstone FA, Levy AP, et al. Screening for Alzheimer's disease by clock drawing. J Am Geriatr Soc 1989;37(8):730–4.

[7] Ferrucci L, Cecchi F, Guralnik JM, et al. Does the Clock Drawing Test predict cognitive decline in older persons independent of the Mini-Mental State Examination? The FINE Study Group. Finland, Italy, The Netherlands Elderly. J Am Geriatr Soc 1996;44(11):1326–31.

[8] Esteban-Santillan C, Praditsuwan R, Ueda H, et al. Clock drawing test in very mild Alzheimer's disease. J Am Geriatr Soc 1998;46(10):1266–9.

[9] Rouleau I, Salmon DP, Butters N, et al. Quantitative and qualitative analyses of clock drawings in Alzheimer's and Huntington's disease. Brain Cogn 1992;18(1):70–87.

[10] Royall DR, Mulroy AR, Chiodo LK, et al. Clock drawing is sensitive to executive control: a comparison of six methods. J Gerontol B Psychol Sci Soc Sci 1999;54B(5):328–33.

[11] Rouleau I, Salmon DP, Butters N. Longitudinal analysis of clock drawing in Alzheimer's disease patients. Brain Cogn 1996;31(1):17–34.

[12] Freund B, Gravenstein S, Ferris R. Use of the Clock Drawing Test as a screen for driving competency in older adults. J Am Geriatr Soc 2002;50(4):S3.

[13] Freedman M, Kaplan E, Delis D, et al. Clock drawing: a neuropsychological analysis. New York: Oxford University Press; 1994.

[14] Tombaugh TN, McDowell I, Krisjansson B, Hubley AM. Mini-Mental State Examination (MMSE) and the Modified MMSE (3MS): a psychometric comparison and normative data. Psychol Assess 1996;8:48–59.

[15] O'Rourke N, Tuokko H, Hayden S, Beattie BL. Early identification of dementia: predictive validity of the clock test. Arch Clin Neuropsychol 1997;12:257–67.

[16] Barr A, Benedict R, Tune L, Brandt J. Neuropsychological differentiation of Alzheimer's disease from vascular dementia. Int J Geriatr Med 1992;7:621–7.

[17] Cahn DA, Salmon DP, Butters N, Wiederholt WC, Corey-Bloom J, Edelstein SL, et al. Detection of dementia of the Alzheimer type in a population-based sample: neuropsychological test perfeormance. J Int Neuropsychol Soc 1995;1:252–60.

[18] Yesavage JA, Brink TL, Rose TL, Lum O, Huang V, Adey MB, et al. Development and validation of a geriatric depression rating scale: a preliminary report. J Psych Res 1983;17:37–49.

[19] World Health Organization. The public health aspects of the aging population. Copenhagen: World Health Organization; 1959.

[20] Knopman DS, Berg JD, Thomas R, Grundman M, Thal LJ, Sano M. Nursing home placement is related to dementia progression: experience from a clinical trial. Alzheimer's disease cooperative study. Neurology 1999;52:714–8.

[21] Williams JH, Drinka TJK, Greenberg JR, Farrell-Holten J, Euhardy R, Schram M. Development and testing of the assessment of living skills and resources (ALSAR) in elderly community dwelling veterans. Gerontologist 1991;31(1):84–91.

[22] Applegate W, Blass J, Williams T. Instruments for the functional assessment of older adults. N Engl J Med 1990;322:1207–14.

[23] Lawton MP, Brody EM. Assessment of older people: self-maintaining and instrumental activities of daily living. Gerontologist 1969;9:179–86.

[24] Katz S, Ford AB, Moskowitz RW, Jackson BA, Jaffe MW. Studies of illness in the aged. The Index of ADL: a standardized measure of biological and social function. JAMA 1963;185:914–9.

[25] Katz S, Downs TD, Cash HR, Gratz RC. Progress in development of the index of ADL. Gerontologist 1970;10:20–30.

[26] Sager MA, Dunham NC, Schwantes A, Mecum L, Halverson K, Harlowe D. Measurement of activities of daily living in hospitalized elderly: a comparison of self-report and performance-based methods. J Am Geriatr Soc 1992;40:457–62.

[27] Inouye SK, van Dyck CH, Alessi CA, Balkin S, Siegal AP, Horwitz RI. Clarifying confusion: the confusion assessment method. A new method for detection of delirium. Ann Intern Med 1990; 113(12):941–8.

[28] Hazzard WR, Blass JP, Hatter JB, Ouslander JG, Tinetti ME. Principles of geriatric medicine and gerontology. 5th edition. New York: McGraw-Hill; 2003.

[29] Freund B, Szinovacz ME. Effects of cognition on driving involvement among the oldest old: variations by gender and alternative transportation opportunities. Gerontologist 2002; 42(5):621–33.

[30] Boustani M, Peterson B, Hanson L, Harris R, Lohr KN. Screening for dementia in primary care: a summary of the evidence for the US Preventive Services Task Force. Ann Intern Med 2003; 138(11):927–37.

ELSEVIER
SAUNDERS

Clin Geriatr Med 20 (2004) 15–25

CLINICS IN
GERIATRIC
MEDICINE

Mild cognitive impairment

David A. Bennett, MD

Rush Alzheimer's Disease Center, Rush University Medical Center, Armour Academic Center, 600 South Paulina, Suite 1028, Chicago, IL 60612, USA

Loss of memory with advanced age has been recognized for more than 4000 years. One of the earliest descriptions can be found in the Precepts of Ptah-hotep. Ptah-hotep was vizier under the reign of Jedkare Isesi, the eighth king of ancient Egypt's fifth Dynasty (c.2414–2375 BCE). In reference to aging, Ptah writes "...the progress of age changes into senility. Decay falls upon a man and decline takes the place of youth. A vexation weighs upon him every day; sight fails, the ear becomes deaf; his strength dissolves without ceasing. The mouth is silent, speech fails him; the mind decays, remembering not the day before" [1]. Thus, memory loss has long been ascribed to the aging process. However, people have also always lived to extreme old age without severe memory loss. For example, although little detail is available regarding the final years of his reign, Pepi II, the last king of the 6th Dynasty, reportedly ruled Egypt for more than 90 years (c.2278–2184 BCE) and lived to the age of 100. By contrast, Dr. Alois Alzheimer published his observations of Auguste D less than 100 years ago. He described the case of a 51-year-old woman with progressive memory impairment, disorientation, aphasia, jealously, paranoia, and hallucinations, who died after a 4-year illness [2]. These anecdotes illustrate the marked heterogeneity of cognitive abilities among older persons, whereby some people can live to extreme old age with little, if any, loss of cognition and others can suffer severe and progressive cognitive decline decades earlier. Thus, before explicitly addressing the issue of mild cognitive impairment (MCI), we must first ask the question: is it normal to lose cognitive function with age? Our expectation of "normal" aging will play a large part in determining what is or is not MCI.

This article was supported by grants from the National Institute on Aging AG10161, AG14449, AG15819.

E-mail address: dbennett@rush.edu

doi:10.1016/j.cger.2003.10.001

Aging and cognitive function

If one uses the term normal to mean typical, usual, or average (in the statistical sense), then there is little doubt that older people perform worse than younger people on a variety of cognitive function tests. Perhaps the most important study examining the relation of age to cognition is the 1955 standardization of the Wechsler Adult Intelligence Scale (WAIS) [3]. This cross-sectional study (in which people of different ages are examined at one time) showed what appeared to be an inexorable decline in cognition beginning in the third decade of life. Before that time, intelligence quotients were being calculated be dividing the "mental age" score by chronologic age. Although this worked well to identify children whose cognition was not maturing appropriately and were in need of additional services, the results were not interpretable when applied to adults or older people as mental age reached an asymptote and chronologic age continued to rise. The solution was to develop normative data for each specific age group and compare an individual's performance with the average performance of his or her age-matched peers. Although the authors were concerned about cohort effects (people born in different decades have markedly different experiences with regard to public health, medical services, and educational resources), they were thought to be small relative to the age-related changes.

As the population aged and dementia became a public health priority, population-based normative data were generated for a variety of dementia screening tests [4,5]. A major problem in using these data for determining "normal" aging was that the samples included older people with age-related diseases. This led to defining normal as typical or usual in the absence of clinical disease. The practice of using age- and education-adjusted normative data from people without clinical disease to inform the diagnosis of dementia achieved rapid and widespread acceptance and remains a standard practice in the neuropsychologic assessment of older people [6–8]. Despite the widespread use of this approach, it has several problems and leads to some counterintuitive conclusions. First, common experience indicates that many older people can reach advanced age without cognitive deterioration. In other words, loss of cognition with age is not inevitable—it is just common. Second, many diseases, especially age-related neurodegenerative diseases, occur slowly over time with long preclinical periods. Thus, the absence of clinical disease cannot necessarily be taken as evidence of the absence of the underlying disease process. For example, the absence of a history of myocardial infarction does not exclude the presence of coronary artery disease. Finally, the use of age-adjusted normative data means that the older you are, the worse your cognitive function needs to be to meet criteria for dementia. This leads to the peculiar conclusion that age protects you from developing dementia. To the extent that age is a proxy for a host of common chronic diseases, one would expect that age would lower the threshold for dementia.

Over the past decade, longitudinal studies have convincingly demonstrated that many, if not most, older people maintain their scores on cognitive function tests over several years of follow-up, even the oldest old [9–11]. This is not to say that older people do not experience subtle cognitive changes. Rather, for most people, those subtle cognitive changes do not manifest as poor scores on cognitive function tests. For example, in one study of a random sample of older people from a geographically defined community population, there was little evidence of cognitive decline among people free of dementia over a period longer than 4 years [9]. Another study of more than 700 older Catholic clergy members without dementia followed for up to 6 years showed marked heterogeneity of cognitive decline with some persons declining precipitously, although most showed little or no decline, and some actually improved [10]. Together these data suggest that measurable cognitive decline in older people is not usual or typical. The decline should be considered in the context of the premorbid level of function rather than the performance of age-matched peers. Cognitive decline likely indicates the presence of a disease process and should be taken seriously.

Definition of mild cognitive impairment

Older people display a spectrum of cognitive abilities that range from cognition little different than that of younger people, to mild impairment, to clinical dementia [10], even at extreme old age [12]. This clinical heterogeneity has been recognized for several decades. The term "benign senescent forgetfulness" was introduced in 1962 to distinguish individuals with mild, minimally progressive cognitive impairment from those with more malignant and progressive dementia [13]. In 1986, a National Institute of Mental Health workshop proposed criteria for age-associated memory impairment [14]. These criteria referred to older persons with mnemonic complaints and documented memory impairment relative to young, healthy adults. The term "mild cognitive impairment" appeared in the literature for the first time in a 1990 publication to refer to people with mild difficulties on cognitive testing but not necessarily distinguishable from mild dementia [15]. This blurring between MCI and mild dementia has continued in some circles. For example, the Clinical Dementia Rating is an instrument in common use to stage dementia [16]. It is scored from 0 (normal) to 3 (advanced dementia). A Clinical Dementia Rating score of 0.5 has been used in some publications to refer to mild dementia [17], while referring to MCI [18] or age-associated memory impairment [19] in other studies. Although this blurring is unlikely to have profound implications for patient evaluation and care, it makes it difficult to interpret the results of the research studies.

Most people now use the term MCI to refer to people with evidence of cognitive impairment on neuropsychologic testing who do not meet criteria for dementia [20–22]. A somewhat less aesthetically pleasing term with a comparable meaning is "cognitively impaired not demented" [23]. Interest in the border zone between normal cognition and mild dementia has increased markedly since the approval of pharmacotherapy for the symptomatic treatment of Alzheimer's disease in the late 1990s, resulting in an international meeting on current Concepts in Mild Cognitive Impairment which was convened in Chicago,

Illinois, in June of 1999 to summarize the clinical, epidemiologic, and pathologic literature [24].

Despite the explosion of interest in MCI over the past few years, there is no consensus regarding its precise definition. This is due to several factors. First, MCI is a heterogeneous condition and does not constitute a distinct disease entity. Although MCI is frequently the earliest clinical manifestation of Alzheimer's disease, other common conditions that cause dementia are also likely to manifest a prodromal or preclinical phase. Thus some investigators require deficits in episodic memory resulting in a condition called amnestic MCI [21], whereas other investigators allow for subtle deficits in multiple domains or a single significant deficit in a domain other than episodic memory [22,25,26]. A second problem is that cognitive performance tests are typically used to document cognitive impairment in MCI [21,22]. The ability to apply cognitive performance tests in a uniform and structured manner is a strength supporting their use for research studies and clinical practice. However, cognitive performance tests are subject to practice effects and random variability [10]. These factors likely contribute to the fact that clinical classification of MCI tends to be an unstable diagnostic category [27]. A third problem relates to the common use of age-adjusted cutoff scores on cognitive function tests when making a diagnosis of MCI as already discussed in detail [21]. This approach artificially truncates the occurrence of the condition because only a limited number of people can fall below the cutoff points and meet criteria for the condition.

Although researchers in the field wrestle with these and other specifics of MCI, there is widespread conceptual agreement that MCI describes older people whose memory or other cognitive abilities are clearly not at the same ability as when they were younger, in whom some impairment can be documented, but who do not meet criteria for dementia. Clinically, the concept is useful because there are many patients who meet these general criteria; patients who have clearly experienced a meaningful and tangible decline in cognition, yet the treating physician may be reluctant to label them as having a dementia. In addition, as will be discussed later, the condition is common and associated with significant morbidity and mortality, making it much more than a theoretical construct. From a research agenda, the concept is useful because it allows intervention in the dementia process at a much earlier stage of disease. Although it is beyond the scope of this review to advocate for any particular set of criteria for MCI, some practical recommendations will be presented in a later section.

Mild cognitive impairment is common

Data are limited on the incidence of (occurrence of new onset disease) MCI with most published studies having too few subjects to draw definitive conclusions. By contrast, slightly more is known about the prevalence of MCI. Reported prevalences range widely and depend, in large part, on the criteria being used and whether one adjusts cognitive test scores for age. For example the

Indianapolis Health and Aging Study reported an overall prevalence of ~ 25% among older persons for cognitive impairment, no dementia, and found that its occurrence increased with age [28]. A slightly lower, but still high prevalence of > 15% among older people was reported previously for the Canadian Health and Aging Study [29]. By contrast, a recent Finnish study reported a prevalence of only ~ 5% [30] and the Leipzig Longitudinal Study of the Aged reported < 5%, although it was as high as 20% if alternate criteria were used [31].

Consequences of mild cognitive impairment

Mortality, institutionalization, and disability

Interest in MCI is also associated with significant morbidity and mortality. Several studies report that people with MCI are about twice as likely to die over the next several years as people without cognitive impairment [32–35]. Further, they appear to be at twofold to threefold increased risk of nursing home placement [12,33]. People with MCI are more impaired on measures of activities of daily living [36] and have greater difficulties managing financial affairs [25]. Together, these data on morbidity and mortality suggest that the condition has a significant impact on clinical milestones important to the lives of patients and their families and their ability to live independently in the community.

Risk of Alzheimer's disease and cognitive decline

Alzheimer's disease develops slowly over many years. Thus, all persons with Alzheimer's disease must have progressed, at some point, through a phase of MCI. A question of great interest is the extent to which MCI represents the beginning of a progressive condition that will develop into full-blown Alzheimer's disease. Numerous studies have examined rates of the development of Alzheimer's disease and other dementias among people with MCI. Crude rates for the development of dementia and Alzheimer's disease from MCI range from < 5% to > 35% per year compared with people without cognitive impairment who developed Alzheimer's disease at rates of 1% to 7% per year [37–41]. Overall, the risk of dementia appears to be increased between threefold and eightfold [22,33,42].

Predictors of Alzheimer's disease and cognitive decline

Because people with MCI clearly seem to be at higher risk for Alzheimer's disease, numerous studies have sought to identify factors that predict the development of Alzheimer's disease among people with MCI. Reported clinical predictors include the presence of functional impairment by self-report or informant report [43] and olfactory deficits [44]. Neuroimaging predictors include the volume of the hippocampus and entorhinal cortex on structural MRI [45,46], reduced glucose metabolism (rCMRGlu) in the temporoparietal region on PET scan [47]. Several studies have examined the ability of cerebrospinal fluid levels of τ- or β-amyloid to predict progression from MCI to Alzheimer's disease; however, the samples in these studies have been too small to draw definitive conclusions [48–50].

Findings from the Religious Orders Study

Several recent studies have taken advantage of clinical data and brain tissue from the Religious Orders Study to examine the clinical and pathologic features of MCI. The Religious Orders Study performs annual clinical evaluations on 1000 older nuns, priests, and brothers from across the country who agreed to organ donation at death. Although people in the study are free of known dementia at entry, many have MCI, and others have developed MCI and Alzheimer's disease since the study began. Details of the clinical and postmortem evaluation can be found in previous publications [10,22,51,52].

Clinical features

The diagnosis of MCI in the Religious Orders Study follows a three-stage process [22]. First, all subjects undergo formal neuropsychologic testing. Second, the test scores are reviewed by a neuropsychologist who determines whether the person has cognitive impairment. Finally, a physician evaluates each participant and determines the presence of dementia. MCI refers to those individuals rated as cognitively impaired by the neuropsychologist but not demented by the examining physician.

We examined risk of death and Alzheimer's disease, and change in cognitive function in more than 200 people with MCI and nearly 600 without cognitive impairment whom we followed for nearly 5 years [22]. People with MCI scored lower on all cognitive tests. They were nearly twice as likely to die and more than three times as likely to develop Alzheimer's disease, in analyses adjusted for age, sex, and education. Finally, they declined faster on measures of episodic memory, language, and cognitive speed but not measures of attention or visuospatial ability.

We also examined the pathologic features of MCI. In one study using a common silver stain to identify classic neuritic plaques and neurofibrillary tangles, all people with MCI proximate to death had some evidence of the pathology of Alzheimer's disease and nearly 40% met accepted pathologic criteria for Alzheimer's disease [53]. Neuritic plaques and neurofibrillary tangles are made up of extracellular deposits of β-amyloid and abnormally phosphorylated intracellular τ proteins. People with MCI had intermediates amounts of amyloid [54] and tangles identified with antibodies to τ [55,56]. Finally, they also had evidence of neuronal loss [57]. Together, these data suggest that in many cases, MCI represents the earliest manifestations of Alzheimer's disease.

Clinical diagnosis of mild cognitive impairment

The data reviewed thus far should make it clear that MCI is common and is associated with significant morbidity and mortality. Thus, despite the absence of commonly accepted criteria and procedures to diagnose MCI, it is incumbent upon each physician to develop some strategy to identify people with the condition. Just like blood pressure is assessed and the heart and lungs auscultated on a regular basis, a brief assessment of brain function should be part of every clinical evaluation. It needn't take more than a few minutes and can easily be incorporated into the general medical examination. The review of systems should include questions for the patient, family member, or both regarding changes in cognition over the past few years. A few brief questions about instrumental activities of daily living such as paying the bills, shopping, cooking, and driving should be asked. The examination should include a general assessment of global cognition. Much of this is already obtained as part of the history. Is the patient able to give a coherent history, in proper sequence, without evidence of word-finding difficulty? Is the patient able to follow directions and take medications without assistance. A brief assessment of delayed recall can easily be incorporated into the exam. For example, show the patient five objects and ask him to recall them after a delay of at least a few minutes. The objects need to be put away afterward so the patient will use recall rather than recognition memory (and the physician needs to remember to ask again after the delay). This combination of memory complaints, general cognitive testing, and delayed recall has been reported to predict the subsequent development of dementia [58]. Significant changes in cognition or daily function not entirely attributable to co-morbidities should make the physician suspicious of cognitive impairment and consider further testing.

Clinical recommendations

The American Academy of Neurology recently developed practice parameters for the detection of MCI [59] and the treatment of dementia [60]. This evidence-based medicine review can make three levels of recommendations: standard (high degree of clinical certainty), guideline (moderate degree of clinical certainty), and option (little empirical support). The report recommended that patients with MCI be identified by clinical evaluation and followed up clinically due to their increased risk of developing dementia (guideline). Using general cognitive screening instruments to aid detection and follow-up (guideline) is also recommended, although brief, focused neuropsychologic test batteries could be considered when screening for dementia (option). It did not address the role of specific neuroimaging procedures or other biologic markers in the detection and follow-up of people with MCI. Thus, these procedures should be considered experimental. The practice parameter on MCI also did not address the use of pharmacologic or nonpharmacologic interventions for MCI. However, the practice parameter for the management of dementia explicitly stated that there is insufficient evidence at this time to recommend the use of cholinesterase inhibitor therapy or other agents used to treat Alzheimer's disease for people with MCI.

Ongoing clinical trials

Several ongoing clinical trials, funded by the National Institutes of Health or pharmaceutical companies, are evaluating the safety and efficacy of various agents in people with MCI to delay progression to Alzheimer's disease. The agents include cholinesterase inhibitor therapy, dopamine agonists, anti-inflammatory agents, vitamin E, ginkgo biloba, and cognitive enhancement training. The results of these trials will become available over the next few years. Further, as agents are developed that slow the progression of Alzheimer's disease, they will logically be tried in MCI to see if they will delay the onset of clinically overt dementia. More information regarding ongoing clinical trials can be obtained from the website: http://www.ClinicalTrials.gov sponsored as a service by the National Institutes of Health through the National Library of Medicine or through the Alzheimer's disease clinical trials database sponsored by the Alzheimer's Disease Education & Referral Center (ADEAR) website: http://www.alzheimers.org/trials sponsored as a service by the National Institute of Aging (1-800-438-4380).

Summary

Interest in the continuum from normal cognition, to MCI, to early Alzheimer's disease has increased considerably since the approval of pharmacologic agents for the symptomatic treatment of Alzheimer's disease. This trend is likely to continue over the next several years as the research community hopes to develop agents for the primary and secondary prevention of Alzheimer's disease. Although no consensus regarding specific clinical criteria for MCI exists, there is general agreement regarding its conceptualization, namely cognitive impairment in the absence of dementia. Data suggest that MCI is common and associated with significant mortality and morbidity. It also appears to be due, in large part, to the same pathologic processes responsible for other age-related dementias, especially Alzheimer's disease, suggesting that public health burden of these conditions is probably much greater than currently recognized. There are no current recommendations regarding specific treatment for MCI. However, a number of clinical trials are underway and data should be forthcoming over the next several years. Future studies are likely to emphasize the identification of risk factors for MCI. Although some data suggest that risk factors for MCI are likely to be similar to those for Alzheimer's disease, this is far from certain, and rigorous, large, longitudinal population-based studies will be required to identify risk factors.

References

[1] Halsall P, editor. Internet ancient history sourcebook. Available at: http://www.fordham.edu/halsall/ancient/ptahhotep.html. Accessed November 28, 2003.
[2] Alzheimer A. A characteristic disease of the cerebral cortex. In: Bick K, Amaducci L, Pepeu G, editors. The early story of Alzheimer's disease. Padova, Italy: Liviana Editrice spa; 1987. p. 1–3.
[3] Wechsler D, editor. The measurement and appraisal of adult intelligence. 4th edition. Baltimore, MD: Williams & Wilkins; 1958.
[4] Crum RM, Anthony JC, Bassett SS, Folstein MF. Population-based norms for the Mini-Mental State Examination by age and educational level. JAMA 1993;269:2386–91.
[5] Williams JG, Huppert FA, Matthews FE, Nickson J. Cognitive Function MRC and Ageing Study (MRC CFAS). Performance and normative values of a concise neuropsychological test (CAMCOG) in an elderly population sample. Int J Geriatr Psychiatry 2003;18:631–44.
[6] Welsh KA, Butters N, Mohs RC, et al. Consortium to Establish a Registry for Alzheimer's Disease (CERAD). Part V. A normative study of the neuropsychological battery. Neurology 1994;44:609–14.
[7] Ganguli M, Ratcliff G, Huff FJ, et al. Effects of age, gender, and education on cognitive tests in a rural elderly community sample: norms from the Monongahela Valley Independent Elders Survey. Neuroepidemiology 1991;10:42–52.
[8] Lucas JA, Ivnik RJ, Smith GE, et al. Normative data for the Mattis Dementia Rating Scale. J Clin Exp Neuropsychol 1998;20:536–47.
[9] Wilson RS, Beckett LA, Bennett DA, Albert M, Evans DA. Change in cognitive function among older persons from a community population: relation to age and Alzeimer's disease. Archives of Neurology 1999;56:1274–9.
[10] Wilson RS, Beckett LA, Barnes LL, et al. Individual differences in rates of change in cognitive abilities of older persons. Psychol Aging 2002;17:179–93.
[11] Howieson DB, Camicioli R, Quinn J, et al. Natural history of cognitive decline in the old old. Neurology 2003;60:1489–94.
[12] Boeve B, McCormick J, Smith G, et al. Mild cognitive impairment in the oldest old. Neurology 2003;60:477–80.
[13] Kral VA. Senescent forgetfulness: benign and malignant. Can Med Assn J 1962;86:257–60.
[14] Crook T, Bartus RT, Ferris SH, et al. Age-associated memory impairment: Proposed diagnostic criteria and measures of clinical change. Dev Neuropsychol 1986;2:261–76.
[15] Jonker C, Hoyer C. The Amstel project: design and first findings. The course of mild cognitive impairment of the aged; a longitudinal 4-year study. Psychiatr J Univ Ott 1990;15:207–11.
[16] Morris JC. The Clinical Dementia Rating (CDR): current version and scoring rules. Neurology 1993;43:2412–4.
[17] Price JL, Morris JC. Tangles and plaques in nondemented aging and "preclinical" Alzheimer's disease. Ann Neurol 1999;45:358–68.
[18] Morris JC, Storandt M, Miller JP, et al. Mild cognitive impairment represents early-stage Alzheimer disease. Arch Neurol 2001;58:397–405.
[19] Goldman WP, Morris JC. Evidence that age-associated memory impairment is not a normal variant of aging. Alzheimer Dis Assoc Disord 2001;15:72–9.
[20] Flicker C, Ferris SH, Reisberg B. Mild cognitive impairment in the elderly: Predictors of dementia. Neurology 1991;41:1006–9.
[21] Petersen RC, Smith GE, Waring SC, Ivnik RJ, Tangalos EG, et al. Mild cognitive impairment: clinical characterization and outcome. Archives of Neurology 1999;56:303–8.

[22] Bennett DA, Wilson RS, Schneider JA, et al. Natural history of mild cognitive impairment in older persons. Neurology 2002;59:198–205.
[23] Ebly EM, Hogan DB, Parhad IM. Cognitive impairment in the nondemented elderly. Results from the Canadian Study of Health and Aging. Arch Neurol 1995;52:612–9.
[24] Petersen RC, Doody R, Kurz A, et al. Current concepts in mild cognitive impairment. Arch Neurol 2001;58:1985–92.
[25] Griffith HR, Belue K, Sicola A, et al. Impaired financial abilities in mild cognitive impairment: a direct assessment approach. Neurology 2003;60:449–57.
[26] Mapstone M, Steffenella TM, Duffy CJ. A visuospatial variant of mild cognitive impairment: getting lost between aging and AD. Neurology 2003;60:802–8.
[27] Ritchie K, Artero S, Touchon J. Classification criteria for mild cognitive impairment: a population-based validation study. Neurology 2001;56:37–42.
[28] Unverzagt FW, Gao S, Baiyewu O, et al. Prevalence of cognitive impairment: data from the Indianapolis Study of Health and Aging. Neurology 2001;57:1655–62.
[29] Graham JE, Rockwood K, Beattie BL, et al. Prevalence and severity of cognitive impairment with and without dementia in an elderly population. Lancet 1997;349:1793–6.
[30] Hanninen T, Hallikainen M, Tuomainen S, Vanhanen M, Soininen H. Prevalence of mild cognitive impairment: a population-based study in elderly subjects. Acta Neurol Scand 2002;106: 148–54.
[31] Busse A, Bischkopf J, Riedel-Heller SG, Angermeyer MC. Mild cognitive impairment: prevalence and incidence according to different diagnostic criteria. Results of the Leipzig Longitudinal Study of the Aged (LEILA75 +). Br J Psychiatry 2003;182:449–54.
[32] Storandt M, Grant EA, Miller JP, Morris JC. Rates of progression in mild cognitive impairment and early Alzheimer's disease. Neurology 2002;59:1034–41.
[33] Tuokko H, Frerichs R, Graham J, et al. I. Five-year follow-up of cognitive impairment with no dementia. Arch Neurol 2003;60:577–82.
[34] Gussekloo J, Westendorp RGJ, Remarque EJ, Lagaay AM, Heeren TJ, Knook DL. Impact of mild cognitive impairment on survival in very elderly people: cohort study. Br Med J 1997;315: 1053–4.
[35] Frisoni GB, Fratiglioni L, Fastbom J, Viitanene M, Winblad B. Mortality in nondemented subjects with coginitive impairment: the influence of health-related factors. Am J Epidemiol 1999;150:1031–44.
[36] Artero S, Touchon J, Ritchie K. Disability and mild cognitive impairment: a longitudinal population-based study. Int J Geriatr Psychiatry 2001;16:1092–7.
[37] Tierney MC, Szalai JP, Snow WG, et al. Prediction of probable Alzheimer's disease in memory-impaired patients: a prospective longitudinal study. Neurology 1996;46:661–5.
[38] Flicker C, Ferris SH, Reisberg B. Mild cognitive impairment in the elderly: predictors of dementia. Neurology 1991;41:1006–9.
[39] Devanand DP, Folz M, Gorlyn M, Moeller JR, Stern Y. Questionable dementia: clinical course and predictors of outcome. J Am Geriatr Soc 1997;45:321–8.
[40] Daly E, Zaitchik D, Copeland M, Schmahmann J, Gunther J, Albert M. Predicting conversion to Alzheimer disease using standardized clinical information. Arch Neurol 2000;57:675–80.
[41] Bowen J, Teri L, Kukull W, McCormick W, McCurry SM, Larson EB. Progression to dementia in patients with isolated memory loss. Lancet 1997;349:763–5.
[42] Larrieu S, Letenneur L, Orgogozo JM, et al. Incidence and outcome of mild cognitive impairment in a population-based prospective cohort. Neurology 2002;59:1594–9.
[43] Tabert MH, Albert SM, Borukhova-Milov L, et al. Functional deficits in patients with mild cognitive impairment: prediction of AD. Neurology 2002;58:758–64.
[44] Devanand DP, Michaels-Marston KS, Liu X, et al. Olfactory deficits in patients with mild cognitive impairment predict Alzheimer's disease at follow-up. Am J Psychiatry 2000;157: 1399–405.
[45] Dickerson BC, Goncharova I, Sullivan MP, et al. MRI -derived entorhinal and hippocampal atrophy in incipient and very mild Alzheimer's disease. Neurobiol Aging 2001;22:747–54.

[46] Jack Jr CR, Petersen RC, Xu YC, et al. Prediction of AD with MRI-based hippocampal volume in mild cognitive impairment. Neurology 1999;52:1397–403.

[47] Arnaiz E, Jelic V, Almkvist O, et al. Impaired cerebral glucose metabolism and cognitive functioning predict deterioration in mild cognitive impairment. Neuroreport 2001;12:851–5.

[48] Riemenschneider M, Lautenschlager N, Wagenpfeil S, Diehl J, Drzezga A, Kurz A. Cerebrospinal fluid tau and beta-amyloid 42 proteins identify Alzheimer disease in subjects with mild cognitive impairment. Arch Neurol 2002;59:1729–34.

[49] de Leon MJ, Segal S, Tarshish CY, et al. Longitudinal cerebrospinal fluid tau load increases in mild cognitive impairment. Neurosci Lett 2002;333:183–6.

[50] Okamura N, Arai H, Maruyama M, et al. Combined Analysis of CSF tau levels and [(123)I]Iodoamphetamine SPECT in mild cognitive impairment: implications for a novel predictor of Alzheimer's disease. Am J Psychiatry 2002;159:474–6.

[51] Schneider JA, Wilson RS, Cochran EJ, et al. Relation of cerebral infarctions to dementia and cognitive function in older person. Neurology 2003;60:1082–9.

[52] Bennett DA, Wilson RS, Schneider JA, et al. Apolipoprotein E4 allele, Alzheimer's disease pathology, and the clinical expression of Alzheimer's disease. Neurology 2003;60:246–52.

[53] DeKosky ST, Ikonomovic M, Styren S, et al. Upregulation of choline acetyltransferase activity in hippocampus and frontal cortex of elderly subjects with mild cognitive impairment. Ann Neurol 2002;51:145–55.

[54] Mufson EJ, Chen EY, Cochran EJ, Beckett LA, Bennett DA, Kordower JH. Entorhinal cortex β-amyloid load in individuals with mild cognitive impairment. Exp Neurol 1999;158:469–90.

[55] Mitchell TW, Mufson EJ, Schneider JA, et al. Parahippocampal tau pathology in healthy aging, mild cognitive impairment and early Alzheimer's disease. Ann Neurol 2002;51:182–9.

[56] Ghoshal N, Garcia-Sierra F, Wuu J, et al. Tau conformational changes correspond to impairments of episodic memory in mild cognitive impairment and Alzheimer's disease. Exp Neurol 2002; 177:475–93.

[57] Kordower JH, Chu Y, Stebbins GT, et al. Loss and atrophy of layer II entorhinal cortex neurons in elderly people with mild cognitive impairment. Ann Neurol 2001;49:202–13.

[58] Palmer K, Backman L, Winblad B, Fratiglioni L. Detection of Alzheimer's disease and dementia in the preclinical phase: population based cohort study. Br Med J 2003;326:245–9.

[59] Petersen RC, Stevens JC, Ganguli M, Tangalos EG, Cummings JL, DeKosky ST. Practice parameter: early detection of dementia: mild cognitive impairment (an evidence-based review). Report of the Quality Standards Subcommittee of the American Academy of Neurology. Neurology 2001;56:1133–42.

[60] Doody RS, Stevens JC, Beck C, et al. Practice parameter: management of dementia (an evidence-based review). Report of the Quality Standards Subcommittee of the American Academy of Neurology. Neurology 2001;56:1154–66.

ELSEVIER
SAUNDERS

Clin Geriatr Med 20 (2004) 27–43

CLINICS IN
GERIATRIC
MEDICINE

Differential diagnosis of dementia syndromes

David S. Geldmacher, MD

Department of Neurology, University of Virginia Health System, P.O. Box 800394, Charlottesville, VA 22908, USA

Many causes of dementia, as well as other syndromes of cognitive impairment, can mimic the clinical state of dementia. Differentiating among these causes is important because of potential differences in symptom management and prognosis. Identifying causes of dementia more precisely is likely to become a prerequisite to initiating disease-specific, long-term, disease-modifying therapy. Nonetheless, the differential diagnosis of dementing conditions can be difficult because of overlap in the clinical expression of quite disparate disease states. Furthermore, the exact pathophysiology of many dementing diseases is controversial, and even the "gold standard" of neuropathologic diagnosis is subject to interpretation.

The construct of dementia

Formally, dementia is a description of a clinical state and does not imply causation or prognosis. In common use, however, dementia is frequently used to describe the underlying brain disease as well as its clinical manifestation. Differentiating the clinical state of dementia from the causative dementing illness is likely to become more important in the future as more treatment options become available. For instance, some treatments might improve the symptoms but not affect the underlying cause of neuronal failure or death. The use of cholinesterase inhibitors in Alzheimer's disease (AD) is the most prevalent example of this type of approach, which is known as symptomatic therapy. In contrast, other treatment approaches may be useful for altering progression of the dementia, but they do not affect the symptoms already present. Using antiplatelet agents or antihypertensives for secondary stroke prevention in patients with vascular dementia is an example of this approach.

E-mail address: dsg8n@virginia.edu

doi:10.1016/j.cger.2003.10.006

Dementia criteria

The diagnosis of dementia generally requires a clinical criterion-matching process. This is necessary because of the numerous causes of dementia (> 60), the lack of clearly defined biomarkers for the common neurodegenerative diseases associated with dementia, and the poor risk-benefit ratio for brain biopsy to obtain tissue for definitive diagnosis when there is no curative therapy available for most dementing illnesses.

The American Academy of Neurology's Practice Parameter for the diagnosis of dementia suggests using the DSM-III-R definition to identify demented individuals in routine clinical practice [1]. The DSM-III-R definition of dementia can be summarized as a state of impaired memory with a loss of other cognitive abilities or change in personality that is persistent (> 6 to 12 months) and interferes with previously achieved levels of social or occupational function [2]. This definition most closely fits the pattern of AD and may not be as easily applied to cognitively disabling brain diseases with memory impairment less prominent than that seen in AD. In general, cognitive changes due to aging, rather than disease, are not functionally disabling.

Cummings and Benson [3] suggested an alternative diagnostic scheme to accommodate the variable expression of memory deficits in dementia syndromes attributable to less common pathologies. Their approach does not require impaired memory to define dementia but depends on the identification of acquired impairment in at least three of the following domains: language, memory, visuospatial skills, emotion/personality, or higher level cognitive functions (abstraction, calculation, judgment, executive function). In further contrast to the DSM-III-R definition, these guidelines do not require the cognitive impairment to be severe enough to interfere with social or occupational function. Similarly, Royall and Polk [4] suggested differentiating dementia syndromes with more diffuse cortical dysfunction, which they denote as Type I dementia, from Type II dementia, which is characterized by relatively greater problems in the execution of complex cognitive tasks (ie, executive dysfunction).

Cortical versus subcortical dementia

The classification of dementia syndromes into "cortical" versus "subcortical" patterns is an older and controversial approach to the clinical diagnostic process. AD is the prototypical cortical dementia, characterized by focal signs of cerebral cortical dysfunction such as semantic language difficulties, visual and spatial disturbances, and apraxia [5]. In contrast, Albert and colleagues [6] defined the typical neuropsychologic pattern of subcortical dementia as a constellation including memory defects, a general slowing of intellectual activity, alterations of personality, and impaired ability to manipulate acquired knowledge. Unlike AD, the memory problems seem to be more in the realm of retrieving information rather than encoding or learning. The cognitive features of subcortical dementia are often seen in association with Parkinsonian motor disorders or other features of basal ganglia (extrapyramidal motor) dysfunction. A weakness of the cortical–subcortical classification is that it does not accurately represent the site of pathology. AD, for instance, is known to have prominent neuronal loss in subcortical structures like the basal forebrain and the locus ceruleus, whereas dementia with Lewy bodies (which frequently expresses the subcortical pattern) is characterized by pathologic findings in cortical neurons. Because of close associations between the frontal lobes and the basal ganglia, frontal cortex lesions may paradoxically produce subcortical cognitive signs. Although subcortical dementia provides a useful shorthand term for communicating a symptom pattern, clinicians should not infer any significant anatomic specificity from its use.

Neuropathologic criteria

The necessity of clinical criteria for dementia classification is underscored by significant controversy about the underlying mechanisms of neuronal dysfunction in the primary degenerative diseases of the brain. Although apparent causative mutations have been found in kindreds with AD and other illnesses, there is no consensus regarding the exact mechanisms by which those mutations lead to cell death. Therefore neuropathologic microscopic diagnosis, typically after autopsy, remains the standard by which clinical diagnostic accuracy is determined. It is important to note however, that there are problems with neuropathologic phenotypic diagnosis. There are for instance, several classification schemes for AD, which could lead one pathologist to make diagnosis of AD and another to implement different criteria and fail to support the diagnosis of AD on the same samples [7]. Even the clear presence of AD pathology may not be associated with a clinical state of dementia [8]. Similar classification problems exist for the pathological diagnosis of dementia with Lewy bodies [9] and frontotemporal dementia [10]. Although it is relatively easy to identify cerebrovascular disease on neuropathologic exam, no uniformly accepted system exists to determine to what extent cerebrovascular lesions contributed to dementia during life.

Identifying potentially reversible sources of dementia

A major goal of the clinical approach to dementia differential diagnosis is the identification of potentially reversible syndromes. These syndromes account for $< 5\%$ of all dementia in most surveys but are not an unusual source of cognitive impairments that do not meet full dementia criteria. Fig. 1 from the United States Federal Agency on Health Care Policy Research [11] illustrates an algorithmic approach to the process of evaluation, emphasizing the importance of aging, delirium, and depression as possible causes of dementia-like symptoms. Bennett, in this issue, addresses age-related cognitive changes and their possible relationship with incipient dementia.

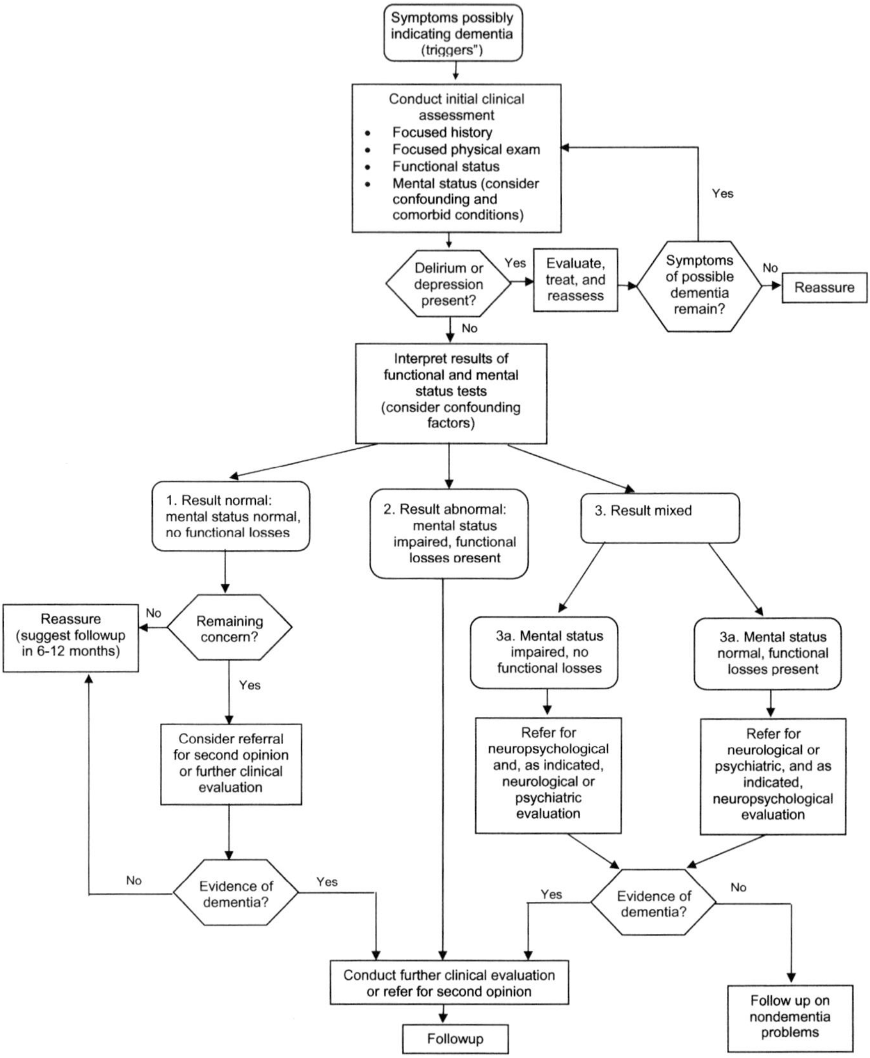

Fig. 1. Flow chart for evaluation of dementia developed by the Agency for Health Care Policy Research (in the public domain) [11].

Dementia versus delirium

Dementia must also be differentiated from delirium in the older adult. Methods to identify delirium are outlined by Freund and Gravenstein in this issue. Delirium is almost always an acute, reversible, and metabolically induced state of fluctuating consciousness. Focal neurologic causes are identified in < 10% older patients with delirium, leading many neurologists to use the term "metabolic encephalopathy" synonymously with delirium. The distinction between delirium and dementia may be hindered by the fact that delirium is a common complication of chronic dementia.

Medications are the most common cause of acutely reversible cognitive impairment [12]. Any drug that affects systemic homeostasis or neuronal function must be considered as a contributing factor to abnormal behavior or cognitive impairment. This is particularly true of drugs intentionally taken for central nervous system (CNS) effects. For example, there was increasing use of diphenhydramine as a nonprescription sedative-hypnotic with age in one recent longitudinal study and a concomitant negative impact on cognitive test scores [13]. If drugs are suspected as a potential contributor, elimination or substitution of agents to avoid cognitive side effects is warranted. Other common causes of delirium in the elderly are fluid and electrolyte derangement, pain, infection, and systemic hypoperfusion (eg, congestive heart failure).

Dementia versus depression

Differentiating irreversible dementia that results from permanent neuronal loss and the potentially reversible cognitive impairments resulting from depression can be problematic, but clinical features can assist with this differentiation. In depression, it is often the patient who complains of cognitive difficulties. In dementia it is usually a relative who brings the patient to the physician. The duration of depression is often shorter, measured in weeks or a few months, and it typically has a more discrete onset than most causes of dementia. A personal or family history of depression also increases the likelihood of depression as a cause of cognitive difficulty. It is unusual for first-ever depression to present after the age of 60 in the absence of a clear precipitant like grieving. Confirming mood changes with the patient is important, because families will often report depression when the actual problem would be better classified as apathy. Apathy is common to both dementia and depression syndromes [14]. Depression rarely leads to focal cognitive deficits like aphasia, apraxia, and agnosia. Patients with depression typically demonstrate psychomotor slowing. The depressed patient often puts forth poor effort or cooperation on cognitive testing and produces incomplete answers with poor effort on testing (eg, "I don't know"). Even when a patient's cognitive function improves with treatment of depression, there is nearly a 50% risk for developing irreversible dementia over the next several years [15].

Other potentially reversible sources of cognitive impairment

This section reviews illness states that may be treated to arrest or reduce progression of dementia. It is important to distinguish "reversible source" from "reversible dementia," because successful treatment of the causative condition may not lead to reversal of symptoms.

Metabolic disturbances

The American Academy of Neurology guidelines for assessment of dementia recommend obtaining blood tests on all patients with suspected dementia to evaluate for potentially reversible causes of cognitive impairment [1]. The recommendation is for clinicians to obtain comprehensive blood chemistry and hematology panels, thyroid function tests, and a vitamin B12 level. Other tests may be useful when there are clinical suspicions, such as sedimentation rate when inflammatory diseases seem likely or heavy metal screening in the context of known or suspected exposures.

Thyroid dysfunction

Most hypothythyroidism in community samples is mild and not associated with significant cognitive impairment [16]. More severe hypothyroidism leads to slowness, inattention, apathy, lethargy, and depression, but frank dementia is uncommon. Psychotic features occur in 3% to 5% of patients with severe hypothyroidism [17]. Only rarely do the cognitive features emerge without the classic systemic features of hypothyroidism.

Hyperthyroidism results in nervousness, irritability, restlessness, hyperkinesia, emotional lability, and inability to concentrate. Confusion and poor performance on cognitive testing may result from reduced ability to focus or concentrate. Paradoxically, depression may be present, but anxiety or mania is more common [18]. As with hypothyroidism, systemic evidence of the disorder is almost always evident when neuropsychiatric manifestations evolve. Neurologic signs, particularly tremor, are frequently present.

Alcohol

Alcohol abuse is often considered as a cause of dementia, but it is unclear that there is a primary alcohol-related dementia. No distinctive pattern of clinical symptoms separates patients with alcohol dementia from alcohol abusers who are not demented [19]. Also, there is no recognized neuropathologic pattern associated with alcoholic dementia. Several syndromes with prominent cognitive deficits have a strong association with alcohol abuse, but these probably act through nutritional deficiencies. They include Korsokoff's syndrome, which is an anterograde amnesia syndrome with a disabling limitation of memory span. It is invariably linked to an acute episode of Wernicke's encephalitis in the context of thiamine deficiency. Patients with Korsokoff's syndrome often cannot retain information in memory for as long as 1 minute and frequently confabulate. Pellagra, the clinical syndrome of nicotinic acid deficiency, also leads to cognitive impairments in alcohol abusers.

Vitamin B12 deficiency

B12 deficiencies can produce a neuropsychiatric syndrome resembling dementia, but the cognitive and behavioral changes usually occur in the context of other neurologic features such as peripheral neuropathy and subacute combined degeneration of the posterior and lateral columns of the spinal cord. Though rare, it is possible for cognitive and behavioral disturbances to occur years before hematologic or spinal cord symptoms appear. Numbness and tingling (parasthesia) in the limbs is the most frequent neurologic symptom. Forgetfulness and irritability are the most common neuropsychiatric features, though psychosis and severe dementia have been seen with protracted B12 deficiency. In patients with neuropsychiatric abnormalities secondary to B12 deficiency, as many as 28% have no anemia or macrocytosis [20]. Complete resolution of dementia with treatment is unusual.

Infection

Cerebral infections can lead to dementia. Herpes simplex virus causes acute hemorrhagic destruction of the memory structures of the mesial temporal lobe. It is rarely mistaken for the degenerative dementias because of its fulminant course and prominent systemic signs of illness. Early treatement with antivirals may prevent death but leave the patient with a persistent amnesia. Fungal infections, in particular cryptococcus, are exceptionally rare causes of cognitive impairments. Both are most commonly seen in patients with immunocompromise. Parasites (eg, toxoplasmosis) can lead to dementia symptoms, often through mass lesions and secondary increases in intracranial pressure. These are identified through cerebral imaging. Because anti-infective therapies are not available for transmissible "prion" diseases, Creutzfeld-Jakob disease will be discussed later.

Syphilis

Dementia caused by syphilis is typically associated with prominent behavioral disturbances, including delusions, emotional lability, hallucinations, and mania. Syphilitic dementia occurs 15 to 30 years after acute exposure. In the pre-antibiotic era, this was a common cause of early-onset dementia, but now late syphilis is sufficiently rare that the most recent evidence-based practice parameters no longer recommend syphilis screening on all dementia cases [1].

When serum markers of syphilis are identified, especially treponemal specific tests, lumbar puncture is indicated. A positive spinal fluid serology is, however, insufficient to diagnose syphilitic dementia, because these markers can remain positive throughout life. Generally, a CSF white blood cell count of $> 5/mm^3$ is necessary to consider a full treatment course of IV antibiotics for neurosyphilis. Dementia should not be expected to resolve, but slowing of progression may be possible.

HIV

Dementia occurs in up to two thirds of individuals with AIDS but is the sole presenting symptom (ie, the AIDS-defining infection or ADI) in $< 10\%$ of cases. The proportion of AIDS dementia as the ADI has been increasing gradually in the era of highly active antiretroviral therapy (HAART), perhaps reflecting that HAART is less effective in controlling the HIV-1 virus in the brain than in other tissues [21]. Psychomotor slowing, inattentiveness, and executive dysfunction are prominent in HIV-related dementia. Focal neurologic signs like ataxia and tremor are often also present. Early treatment of HIV infection may delay or prevent development of severe dementia, and survival is enhanced with HAART [21]. HIV-positive individuals with rapid loss of cognitive function should be assessed for acute cerebral infections, like toxoplasmosis and progressive multifocal leukoencephalopathy.

Reversible vascular disturbances

There is a clear association between cerebral infarction and dementia, which will be addressed later in the section on vascular dementia. There is little experimental support to suggest that there are chronic cognitive deficits related to cerebrovascular insufficiency that does not cause permanent ischemic damage. However, cerebrovascular inflammation is a known reversible source of cognitive impairment. The cerebral vasculitides are a group of disorders of widely disparate causes that may present with cognitive disorders. As with HIV, the systemic illness is apparent before signs of cognitive or behavioral disorder in most individuals. Primary angiitis of the CNS is, however, an extremely rare vasculitic syndrome that presents with dementia. About 30% have cognitive impairment at first presentation [22]. The disorder characterized by progressive cognitive decline over months in the absence of systemic signs. The symptom pattern is dependent on the areas of brain affected by the patchy inflammation but most commonly includes prominent executive function and attention deficits. Primary CNS angiitis may present throughout adult life, without a strong weighting toward the elderly. Diagnosis depends on cerebral angiography and meningeal/brain biopsy.

Anatomic abnormalities

The American Academy of Neurology practice parameter for diagnosis of dementia recommends the use of cerebral imaging as part of the diagnostic process [1]. Scheltens addresses the utility of imaging elsewhere in this issue. Many practitioners use it to identify cerebrovascular burden, but imaging also provides the opportunity to find lesions amenable to surgical intervention. These may be mass lesions like meningioma or subdural hematoma. In the rare cases with these abnormalities, reversal of dementia symptoms may be complete and permanent (though not always).

Hydrocephalus

Normal pressure hydrocephalus (NPH) is another rare form of dementia, but it is potentially reversible by ventriculoperitoneal shunting. It is classically characterized by a triad of gait disorder, urinary incontinence, and cognitive decline but today is most commonly raised as a part of the differential diagnosis by findings on imaging tests. Each of the three clinical elements is relatively common in elderly individuals, and their co-occurrence in the presence of brain atrophy on cerebral imaging is not sufficient for the diagnosis of NPH.

In most patients the gait disorder appears first, followed by the cognitive changes. The gait dysfunction is characterized by short steps and poor turning ability. The gait has been described as "magnetic," and patients may report they feel as though their feet are stuck to the floor. Cognitive symptoms are typically mild and include psychomotor slowing, with impaired concentration and mild memory difficulties. Focal cortical symptoms (such as the aphasia, apraxia, and agnosia characteristic of AD) are exceptionally rare, as is psychosis. Urinary incontinence is variably expressed and may not occur. Because prostatism in men and stress incontinence in women are common in the age groups at risk for NPH, the predictive value of incontinence is low.

A combination of clinical and imaging criteria can be used to predict response to shunting. Beyond these criteria, a positive response to removal of a large volume of spinal fluid by lumbar puncture perhaps remains the best predictor of treatment success with ventriculoperitoneal shunting [23]. It is, however, complicated by a high false-negative rate.

Characterizing progressive dementia syndromes

It is most common for the evaluation for dementia mimics or reversible sources of dementia to prove negative, leading to a diagnosis of progressive, or at least permanent, dementia. This section identifies key aspects of the more common forms of degenerative or progressive dementia. The emphasis will be on the expression of earlier phases of the illnesses, when clinicians are likely to first encounter the problems. Clinical distinctions between chronic dementia states become progressively more difficult with increasing disease severity. A more detailed exploration of the neuropsychologic profiles of these illnesses is covered by Manning elsewhere in this issue.

Alzheimer's disease

Key clinical features of AD are listed in Box 1. The recommended criteria for diagnosing AD incorporate recognizing these cardinal features: (1) insidious onset, (2) progressive course, (3) memory loss, and (4) at least one other focal cognitive disturbance such as language dysfunction, apraxia, visuoperceptual or visuospatial disorder, or executive dysfunction. These impairments should represent a decline from past levels of performance and interfere with usual established patterns of daily function. The motor examination is generally normal. The frequency of AD and its common presentation were sufficient for a consensus panel to recommend that AD be considered a diagnosis of inclusion [24]. It is therefore important to note that the well recognized but relatively insensitive research criteria for AD [25] need not be applied in clinical settings [1,24].

Impediments to diagnosis

Early recognition of AD (as well as other primary degenerative dementias) is made difficult by many factors, especially symptoms that render patients less likely to seek care on their own and reduce their effectiveness as reporters of

Box 1. Key elements of the clinical syndrome in mild AD

Onset

Insidious

Course

Progressive

Cognitive findings

Impaired orientation
Impaired learning and recent memory
Empty speech and anomia
Visuospatial problems

Functional/behavioral findings

Executive dysfunction (may be subtle)
Apathy
Poor self-awareness
Emotional withdrawal

Neurologic exam

No CNS findings

their overall ability. These "negative symptoms" are important, but under-recognized management problems in AD [26,27].

Self-awareness

Many patients with AD do not recognize that they are impaired. This can range from mild denial of functional impairment to frank anosognosia (unawareness of illness). The problem has been linked to difficulty in implicit learning of intellectual limitations [28], rather than a more active psychologic "denial" of illness. In effect, the patients forget that they forget things. They also forget what they forget, so when challenged by professionals or caregivers, people affected by AD may seem surprised that others have recognized a problem. Similarly, AD patients underestimate their impairments across a broad spectrum of cognition and function. There is frequent concurrence of confabulation (ie, fabricating in place of remembering) in conjunction with anosognosia. When unawareness is present, it is an even greater source of distress to families than the overall disease severity [29].

Executive or "frontal lobe" function

Problems with judgment, problem solving, planning, and abstract thought are common in early AD. These problems are frequently masked by or confused with more overt memory problems. Intact executive function requires selecting tasks appropriately, properly sequencing their execution, and monitoring performance to ensure successful completion. Inability to maintain complex goal-directed behaviors results in impersistence at tasks, new or worsened procrastination, poor planning, and impaired problem solving. These become evident as difficulty in handling household paperwork (like insurance policies or even sorting out "junk mail") or as a constriction of everyday skills like meal preparation.

Apathy

Apathy is a lack of motivation or behavioral initiation that is not attributable to disordered consciousness or emotional distress [14]. It is a pervasive problem throughout the course of AD and is perhaps the most common adverse behavior in the illness, with one study reporting a prevalence of 92% [30]. Apathetic behaviors are often misattributed to insensitivity, disinterest, and voluntary or willful refusal to cooperate on the part of the patient [31]. Apathy places excessive demands on caregivers and contributes to a high degree of caregiver distress [32]. Distinguishing apathy from depression can be very difficult for family members and clinicians alike, because both syndromes are associated with anhedonia and a reduction in self-initiated activities.

Passivity and withdrawal

Passive behavioral changes are seen in up to two thirds of patients with mild AD [33]. Patients may also exhibit decreased affectionate behaviors and verbalizations [34]. In many cases, passive personality change long predates cognitive abnormality, but this is only discerned retrospectively. One retrospective review suggested that social withdrawal, mood changes, or depression were present in > 70% of cases, with a mean duration of more than 2 years before diagnosis of AD [35].

Frontotemporal dementia

The understanding of frontotemporal dementia (FTD) has undergone rapid changes in the last 10 years. The classic term Pick's disease has been superseded in clinical use, and FTD is now often considered to consist of three main syndromes: (1) the frontal variant, in which behavioral and judgment changes are most prominent, (2) progressive nonfluent aphasia, and 3) semantic dementia, which is characterized by fluent aphasia with a loss of word knowledge. Either of the aphasic forms may also include elements of executive dysfunction. Criteria for diagnosing this grouping of dementia syndromes have been updated recently [36].

Alzheimer's disease versus frontal variant frontotemporal dementia

In clinical settings, differentiating AD from the frontal form of FTD can be quite difficult when the clinician sees relatively few cases of frontal dementia. Behavioral changes like poor personal and social judgment are its hallmarks. Perseveration and stereotyped behaviors may also be seen. Disordered initiation, goal-setting, and planning (ie, executive dysfunction) are accompanied by apathetic or disinhibited behavior. Most patients have little awareness of these changes and actively deny or refute any problems (anosognosia). Performance on cognitive screening tests, like the Mini-Mental State Examination, is often normal or minimally impaired [37]. This is different from AD, in which this level of behavioral disturbance is usually associated with obviously poor cognitive test scores. Any combination of these symptoms is possible as the illness progresses, and most patients present with a syndrome of sluggishness with apathy, inertia, aspontaneity, punctuated by episodes of disinhibition and stereotyped behaviors [37]. The impaired praxis and visuospatial function characteristic of AD are usually not seen in individuals with frontal dementia until late in the course, if at all.

Dementia with Lewy bodies

Dementia associated with atypical clinical or neuropathologic manifestations of Parkinson's disease has become recognized as a common syndrome. A very confusing nomenclature on this topic was partially resolved by the establishment of clinical criteria using the term "dementia with Lewy bodies" to supersede a myriad of other descriptors including diffuse Lewy body disease and Lewy body variant of AD, among others [38]. This nomenclature implicitly avoids any assumptions of the role of the Lewy bodies as the pathophysiologic cause of the observed dementia. Key features of the clinical syndrome of dementia with Lewy bodies are illustrated in Box 2.

The cognitive/behavioral and Parkinsonian signs typically evolve within 1 year of each other. Disorders of executive function are among the earliest cognitive problems. In contrast to AD, visual hallucinations may become evident early in the course. They may be provoked or exacerbated by attempted treatment of the Parkinsonism. The hallucinations are almost universally benign. Nighttime behavioral disturbances, such as the violent or active dreams characteristic of rapid eye movement (REM) sleep behavioral disturbance, may predate other symptoms [39]. Apathy and depression are also frequent. Some patients experience abrupt fluctuations in awareness. When present, these fluctuations are highly specific for dementia with Lewy bodies.

On examination, visuospatial disturbances are often prominent. Other changes include general slowness of thought and action (bradyphrenia or psychomotor slowing). Rigidity is far more typical than Parkinson's type tremor, affecting

Box 2. Key elements of the clinical syndrome in mild dementia with Lewy bodies

Onset

Insidious

Course

Progressive
Sleep disturbance early (eg, vivid dreams, REM-sleep behavioral disorder, periodic limb movements)

Cognitive findings

Visuospatial problems

Functional/behavioral findings

Executive dysfunction
Visual hallucinations

Neurologic exam

Masked face
Rigidity
(Tremor is unusual)

about 75% of cases. Bradykinesia also appears in a large majority of cases. Unsteady gait and postural instability are typical.

Key features of the dementia with Lewy bodies and other uncommon dementing illnesses that may present with Parkinsonism are illustrated in Table 1.

Vascular dementia

Dementia resulting from cerebrovascular disease, now known as vascular dementia (VaD), is an old observation. The concept of VaD has evolved rapidly in the last decade and continues to be the subject of much nosological debate. It is intuitively obvious that recurrent cerebral infarctions would cause losses of intellectual function. Defining how the infarctions are detected, how much and which parts of the brain are affected, and to what extent classical ischemic infarction is necessary for expression of the syndrome remain problematic. Three broad classes of vascular dementia have been described. These are dementia syndromes due to (1) multiple discrete infarctions, (2) strategic single infarcts, and (3) diffuse subcortical white matter disease. Because vascular risk factors and cerebrovascular disease are common in the age group typically evaluated for

Table 1
Distinguishing features of dementia syndromes associated with prominent Parkinsonian motor dysfunction

	Dementia with Lewy bodies	Parkinson's disease with dementia	Progressive supranuclear palsy	Corticobasal degeneration
Motor symptoms predate dementia (> 1 year)		+	+/–	+
Hallucinations	+	+		
Rigidity	+	+	+ (neck > limbs)	+/–
Lateralized motor symptoms		+		+
Downgaze paralysis			+	
Prominent gait disturbance		+	+	
Unilateral apraxia				+
Lateralized cortical sensory loss				+

dementia, the clinician faces the problem of discerning whether cerebrovascular disease is the sole cause of the cognitive impairments or merely a concomitant or complicating factor. As many as one third of patients with AD pathology may also have cerebrovascular disease present on autopsy. There are no practical criteria to know how much the cerebrovascular disease was contributing to the expression of dementia.

The most specific criteria for the diagnosis of VaD require a temporal association between the cerebrovascular event and the onset of dementia [40]. The presence of scattered or nonconfluent white matter changes on cerebral imaging in a person with gradually progressing dementia is generally insufficient to consider cerebrovascular disease as the sole cause of the impairments. On examination, patients with diffuse subcortical cerebrovascular disease will typically exhibit psychomotor slowing and depressive features, without the anomia or visuospatial impairments characteristic of AD. Patients with discrete infarcts can be expected to have focal neurologic signs consistent with the lesion location (eg, weakness, tone changes, visual field deficits). Many patients with VaD will have gait impairments and urinary changes, which may resemble those seen in hydrocephalus. Common clinical features of VaD are listed in Box 3.

Creutzfeld-Jakob disease

Creutzfeld-Jakob disease (CJD) is the prototypic human disease caused by transmissible proteins known as prions. The classic triad of CJD involves dementia, myoclonus, and a distinctive periodic discharge pattern on electroencephalography. Vague initial symptoms of irritability and unusual somatic sensations occur in about one third of cases. Complex visual dysfunction is a common part of the cognitive loss. The rate of progression distinguishes CJD

Box 3. Typical elements of the clinical syndrome in VaD

Onset

Subtle (common) or abrupt (less common)

Course

Variable

Comorbidities

Hypertension
Diabetes mellitus
Coronary artery disease
Peripheral vascular disease

Cognitive findings

Slowing
Focal cognitive deficits (correlate with lesions on imaging)

Functional/behavioral findings

Urinary incontinence
Executive dysfunction
Depression
Preserved awareness

Neurologic exam

Focal findings (eg, lateralized hyper-reflexia)
Rigidity
Gait disturbance

from nearly all other forms of dementia. Patients exhibit overt changes in cognitive and functional ability from month to month, or even more rapidly. Most patients become akinetic and mute within 6 months of diagnosis and die within one year. Clinical criteria have now been developed to improve diagnostic accuracy [41].

Summary

Differential diagnosis of dementia remains an art demanding of the clinician's skills. The absence of gold standards for diagnosis and the sometimes poor links between clinical disease and neuropathologic findings add to the challenge. Nonetheless, the continued development and updating of both practice parameters and diagnostic criteria provide the practitioner with the background to make informed diagnostic decisions.

References

[1] Knopman DS, DeKosky ST, Cummings JL, et al. Practice parameter: diagnosis of dementia (an evidence-based review). Report of the Quality Standards Subcommittee of the American Academy of Neurology. Neurology 2001;56:1143–53.
[2] American Psychiatric Association. Diagnostic and statistical manual of mental disorders. DSM-III-R. 3rd edition, revised. Washington, DC: American Psychiatric Association; 1987.
[3] Cummings JL, Benson DF. Dementia: a clinical approach. 2nd edition. Boston: Butterworth-Heinemann; 1992.
[4] Royall DR, Polk M. Dementias that present with and without posterior cortical features: an important clinical distinction. J Am Geriatr Soc 1998;46:98–105.
[5] Talwalker S. The cardinal features of cognitive and noncognitive dysfunction and the differential efficacy of tacrine in Alzheimer disease patient. J Biopharm Stat 1996;6:443–56.
[6] Albert ML, Feldman RG, Willis AL. The "subcortical dementia" of progressive supranuclear palsy. J Neurol Neurosurg Psychiatry 1974;37:121–30.
[7] Jobst KA, Barnetson LP, Shepstone BJ. Accurate prediction of histologically confirmed Alzheimer's disease and the differential diagnosis of dementia: the use of NINCDS-ADRDA and DSM-III-R criteria, SPECT, X-ray CT, and Apo E4 in medial temporal lobe dementias. Oxford Project to Investigate Memory and Aging. Int Psychogeriatr 1988;10:271–302.
[8] Goldman WP, Price JL, Storandt M, Grant EA, McKeel DW, Rubin EH, Morris JC. Absence of cognitive impairment or decline in preclinical Alzheimer's disease. Neurology 2001;56:361–7.
[9] Del Ser T, Hachinski V, Merskey H, Munoz DG. Clinical and pathological features of two groups of patients with dementia with Lewy bodies: effect of coexisting Alzheimer-type lesion load. Alzheimer Dis Assoc Disord 2001;15:31–44.
[10] Lund and Manchester Groups. Clinical and neuropathological criteria for frontotemporal dementia. J Neurol Neurosurg Psychiatry 1994;57:416–8.
[11] Costa Jr PT, Williams TF, Somerfeld M, et al. Early identification of Alzheimer's disease and related dementias. Clinical practice guideline, quick reference guide for clinicians, no. 19. Rockville, MD: US Department of Health and Human Services, Public Health Service, Agency for Health Care Policy Research AHCPR Publication No. 97–0703; November 1996.
[12] Clarfield AM. The reversible dementias: do they reverse? Ann Intern Med 1988;109:476–86.
[13] Basu R, Dodge H, Stoehr GP, Ganguli M. Sedative-hypnotic use of diphenhydramine in a rural, older adult, community-based cohort: effects on cognition. Am J Geriatr Psychiatry 2003;11: 205–13.
[14] Landes A, Sperry SD, Strauss ME, Geldmacher DS. Apathy in Alzheimer's disease. J Am Geriatr Soc 2001;49:1700–7.
[15] Alexopolous GS, Meyers BS, Young RC, et al. The course of geriatric depression with "reversible dementia": a controlled study. Am J Psychiatry 1993;150:1693–9.
[16] Lubositzky R, Oberman AS, Kaufman N, Reichman N, Flatau E. Prevalence of cognitive dysfunction and hypothyroidism in an elderly community population. Isr J Med Sci 1996;32: 60–5.
[17] Swanson JR, Kelly JJ, McConahey WM. Neurologic aspects of thyroid dysfunction. Mayo Clin Proc 1981;56:504–12.
[18] Jadresic DP. Psychiatric aspects of hyperthyroidism. J Psychosom Res 1990;34:603–15.
[19] Munro CA, Saxton J, Butters MA. Alcohol dementia: "cortical" or "subcortical" dementia? Arch Clin Neuropsychol 2001;16:523–33.

[20] Lindenbaum J, Healton EB, Savage DG, et al. Neuropsychiatric disorders caused by cobalamine deficiency in the absence of anemia or macrocytosis. N Engl J Med 1988;318:1720–8.
[21] Dore GJ, McDonald A, Li Y, Kaldor JM, Brew BJ. National HIV Surveillance Committee. Marked improvement in survival following AIDS dementia complex in the era of highly active antiretroviral therapy. AIDS 2003;17:1539–45.
[22] Abu Shakra M, Khraishi M, Grosman H, et al. Primary angiitis of the CNS diagnosed by angiography. Q J Med 1994;87:351–8.
[23] Vanneste JAL. Diagnosis and management of normal-pressure hydrocephalus. J Neurol 2000; 247:5–14.
[24] Small GW, Rabins PV, Barry PB, et al. Diagnosis and treatment of Alzheimer's disease and related disorders: consensus statement of the American Association for Geriatric Psychiatry, the Alzheimer's Association, and the American Geriatrics Society. JAMA 1997;278:1363–71.
[25] McKhann G, Drachman D, et al. Clinical diagnosis of Alzheimer's disease: report of the NINCDS-ADRDA work group under the auspices of the Department of Health and Human Services Task Force on Alzheimer's disease. Neurology 1984;34:939–44.
[26] Ott BR, Noto RB, Fogel BS. Apathy and loss of insight in Alzheimer's disease: a SPECT imaging study. J Neuropsychiatr Clin Neurosci 1996;8:41–6.
[27] Reichman WE, Coyne AC, Amireni S, Molino Jr B, Egan S. Negative symptoms in Alzheimer's disease. Am J Psychiatry 1996;153:424–6.
[28] Starkstein SE, Sabe L, et al. Anosognosia and procedural learning in Alzheimer's disease. Neuropsychiatry Neuropsychol Behav Neurol 1997;10(2):96–101.
[29] Seltzer B, Vasterling JJ, et al. Awareness of deficit in Alzheimer's disease: relation to caregiver burden. Geron 1997;37(1):20–4.
[30] Mega MS, Cummings JL, Fiorello T, Gornbein J. The spectrum of behavioral changes in Alzheimer's disease. Neurology 1996;46:130–5.
[31] Campbell JJ, Duffy JD. Treatment strategies in amotivated patients. Psychiatr Ann 1997;27: 44–9.
[32] Greene JG, Smith R, Gardiner M, Timbury GC. Measuring behavioral disturbance of elderly demented patients in the community and its effects on relatives: A factor analytic study. Age Ageing 1982;11:121–6.
[33] Rubin EH, Morris JC, Berg L. The progression of personality changes in senile dementia of the Alzheimer's type. Am Geriatr Soc 1987;35(8):721–5.
[34] Mendez MF, Martin R, et al. Psychiatric symptoms associated with Alzheimer's disease. J Neuropsychiatry Clin Neurosci 1990;2:28–33.
[35] Jost BC, Grossberg GT. The evolution of psychiatric symptoms in Alzheimer's disease: a natural history study. J Am Geriatr Soc 1996;44(9):1078–81.
[36] McKhann GM, Albert MS, Grossman M, et al. Work Group on Frontotemporal Dementia and Pick's Disease. Clinical and pathological diagnosis of frontotemporal dementia: report of the Work Group on Frontotemporal Dementia and Pick's Disease. Arch Neurol 2001;58: 1803–9.
[37] Hodges JR. Frontotemporal dementia (Pick's disease): clinical features and assessment. Neurology 2001;56(Suppl):S6–10.
[38] McKeith IG, Galasko D, Kosaka K, et al. Consensus guidelines for the clinical and pathologic diagnosis of dementia with Lewy bodies (DLB): report of the consortium on DLB international workshop. Neurology 1996;47:1113–24.
[39] Boeve BF, Silber MH, Ferman TJ, et al. REM sleep behavior disorder and degenerative dementia: an association likely reflecting Lewy body disease. Neurology 1998;51:363–70.
[40] Roman GC, Tatemichi TK, Erkinjuntti T, Cummings JL, Masdeu JC, Garcia JH, et al. Vascular dementia: diagnostic criteria for research studies: report of the NINDS-AIREN International Workshop. Neurology 1993;43:250–60.
[41] Brandel JP, Delasnerie-Laupretre N, Laplanche JL, et al. Diagnosis of Creutzfeld Jakob disease:effect of clinical criteria on incidence estimates. Neurology 2000;54:1095–9.

ELSEVIER
SAUNDERS

Clin Geriatr Med 20 (2004) 45–58

CLINICS IN
GERIATRIC
MEDICINE

Beyond memory: neuropsychologic features in differential diagnosis of dementia

Carol Manning, PhD

Department of Neurology, P.O. Box 800394, University of Virginia Health System, Charlottesville, VA 22908-0394, USA

Although the term "dementia" is sometimes used as a synonym for memory loss in general or Alzheimer's disease (AD) in particular, dementia is an umbrella term that describes a constellation of symptoms rather than a specific etiology or disease process. As it is most commonly defined, dementia denotes memory impairment combined with disturbance in at least one other area of cognition (DSM-IV) [1]. This definition best describes patients with medial temporal lobe involvement and may exclude those with pathology in other brain areas. The currently accepted definition of dementia is likely to be revised as understanding of cognitive dementia syndromes and their underlying pathology becomes more sophisticated.

Memory difficulty is among the most common cognitive complaints from patients and caregivers alike when describing patients' cognitive difficulties. Patients are often inexact and attribute difficulties to memory when subsequent cognitive testing reveals that the deficits are in other cognitive domains. Furthermore, although current diagnostic criteria specifically select for memory deficits among those diagnosed with dementia, neuropsychologic testing often reveals significant deficits in other areas of cognition. Using current guidelines (DSM-IV, ICD-9) [1,2], individuals without memory difficulty but with deficits in nonmemory cognition would not be diagnosed with dementia, yet these deficits may have significant impact on everyday functioning and may indicate disease processes.

As noted in a previous article in this issue, dementia does not present with just one profile. Although individual differences in presentation exist, individuals with common underlying dementia pathology most often have striking similarities in presentation. Different dementias have different "signatures" that provide important information regarding the etiology and clinical course of the disease. In

E-mail address: cm4r@virginia.edu

doi:10.1016/j.cger.2003.10.002

addition, clarification of the cognitive profile provides information on pharmacologic and behavioral treatment strategies.

What is neuropsychology?

Clinical neuropsychology is an evidence-based field involving the relationship between brain functioning and behavioral expression. This relationship is viewed in terms of neurocognition and neurobehavior. Neuropsychology relies heavily on quantitative statistical techniques borrowed from the field of psychology [3]. As such, the measurement of neurocognition uses standardized tests with strict and uniform administration and scoring. Test interpretation is based on extensive normative data taking into account age, education, and even cultural factors. Additional normative data are available for individuals with a wide variety of neurologic and other medical conditions. Therefore clear performance expectations exist for most individuals. Neuropsychologists are also concerned with neurobehavior, which involves psychosocial factors resulting from or contributing to brain dysfunction as well as psychosocial factors that mimic brain dysfunction. It is the role of the neuropsychologist to tease apart these factors and understand their impact on the individual.

Most neuropsychologic evaluations involve a clinical interview with the patient. An interview with a spouse or caregiver familiar with the patient is often appropriate, especially if dementia is suspected. The interview is critical to discern important history, clarify qualitative elements of neurobehavioral functioning, and often serves to put the patient at ease. Standardized neurocognitive testing generally follows the interview. The length of time required for the testing is determined by the complexity of the referral question and the performance of the individual.

How neuropsychology can help

Neuropsychologic assessment is designed to provide important information to the referring physician or health care provider and to the patient and family. Common purposes of the neuropsychologic assessment include providing diagnostic information, documentation of change over time, and assessment of treatment efficacy. First, the neuropsychologic assessment provides diagnostic information by revealing patterns of performance in relation to neurodegenerative disease states and identifying patterns of deficits that are referable to particular brain areas of dysfunction. These patterns of deficit generally are easiest to discern earlier in the disease state before global decline occurs.

A good neuropsychologic examination clarifies and documents cognitive difficulties that are missed on bedside examination. The Mini-Mental State Exam (MMSE) [4], a widely used instrument, is useful for detecting dementia in clearly demented individuals but has decreased sensitivity and can miss mild dementia in individuals who are highly educated or who have high premorbid functioning [5,6]. Clinicians should be aware that a high score on the MMSE does not adequately rule out the possibility of dementia or cognitive decline in high-functioning individuals with cognitive complaints. The MMSE generally does not provide sufficient information on the cognitive profile to aid in a specific dementia diagnosis. An additional caveat regarding the use of the MMSE is its insensitivity in demented individuals at the lower end of the spectrum—it does not provide information on relative abilities within people with moderate to severe dementia. Therefore, the MMSE is a useful bedside tool for determining the existence of dementia in average individuals but does not rule out dementia in more educated mildly demented people, and it does not provide detailed cognitive information to aid in diagnosis of specific dementia type.

The neuropsychologic assessment also addresses psychosocial issues that occur both as a consequence of and coincident with the cognitive dysfunction. For example, the presence of depression versus dementia is a common referral question. All too often, the answer is both, particularly early in a dementing process. As will be discussed later, depression has negative impacts on cognition and can cause excess disability if left untreated.

A neuropsychologic assessment can be a resource for patients and families as well as the referring physician. For instance, the differentiation of depression versus apathy is an important caregiver issue. Family members often misperceive apathy as depression, leaving caregivers frustrated and feeling helpless. Differentiation provided by the assessment along with subsequent education can relieve significant guilt and improve family psychosocial functioning. The neuropsychologic assessment also provides information on the patient's capabilities so that patients and families alike help the patient rely on strengths rather than weaknesses.

Cognition

Memory

Without memory we are lost, floating without ties to people and occasions that bring our lives meaning. Memory provides us with context and enables us to guide our behavior by using past experience. Therefore, the loss of memory is highly feared. Extensive memory loss causes extreme disability, whereas mild loss is associated with disorientation and depression.

Memory is hypothesized to involve at least two separate systems involving declarative memory and procedural memory [7–9]. These memory systems are distinct, dissociable, and involve independent neural systems [10]. Declarative memory involves conscious awareness of memory for events, objects, and general recollection or recognition [10]. Declarative memory is highly dependent on the hippocampal formation and thus is severely affected by AD.

Encoding, storage, and retrieval all need to take place within the declarative system for accurate recall to take place. Encoding involves initial registration and learning of the material. Material that is not accurately encoded cannot be recalled. Storage involves retaining a representation of the encoded material for future recall. Memory storage involves physiologic changes at the neuronal level, including dendritic branching and neurotransmission with particular dependence on the cholinergic system [11]. Memory retrieval is the ability to access stored information when needed. Free recall involves remembering the material unaided, whereas recognition involves correctly selecting the stored information from choices. Poor recall with good recognition implies a retrieval deficit rather than a storage deficit.

Recent memory refers to events that happened within a short time period relative to recall. This would include events within the last few weeks and memory for information learned within the testing situation. Remote memory refers to events occurring long ago, usually in childhood or early adulthood.

The second memory system involves procedural memory which is "how to" memory. This includes motor memory for things like riding a bicycle or even remembering a sequence of actions or movements [12]. Procedural memory does not necessitate conscious awareness of an activity, action, or the steps required to accurately perform a task. Procedural memory involves the dorsolateral prefronto-striatal loop and is thus likely to be impaired in individuals with basal ganglia or prefrontal cortex dysfunction [13–16].

Attention

Attention varies over time depending on characteristics of the material at hand such as novelty and complexity. Attention also varies between people depending on variables including age and disease. Sustained attention involves the ability to maintain focus and direction. An important characteristic of attention is limited capacity [17]. Simple attention involves the ability to attend to one set of information with no need to attend to competing distractions. An example of simple attention is the ability to repeat information heard in a quiet room. Divided attention involves attending to two things at once, such as listening to the radio while driving a car. Attention decreases even with healthy aging [18]. Attention does not appear to be localized to a particular brain area and depending on the kind of task has been shown to involve regions of the frontal, parietal, and temporal lobes [19–21].

Praxis

Praxis involves directed coordination of movements. Apraxia involves problems that can not be attributed to the motor system or muscle coordination [22]. Ideomotor apraxia involves knowledge of the desired action with inability to accurately execute the actions. The patient with ideational apraxia has impaired understanding of the action itself and often has difficulty recognizing the use of common objects. The parietal lobes are implicated in apraxia involving loss of skilled movements [23].

Language

Intact language ability has many components including expression, reception, and repetition; each is associated with particular brain areas and associated aphasias. Expression difficulties with relatively intact comprehension are localized to Broca's area [24]. Comprehension deficits with fluent but muddled speech are associated with Wernicke's area [24]. Language deficits can mask or magnify underlying memory difficulties. Neuropsychologic examination of language provides diagnostic information regarding not only the nature of language deficits but also the existence of deficits in other areas difficult to assess because of language problems.

Executive functioning

Executive functioning is becoming recognized as critical in the understanding of dementia. Executive functioning involves uniquely human abilities including abstraction, planning for the future, development of novel ideas, using feedback to guide performance, sequencing, and the ability to "switch set" from one idea to another. Deficits in executive functioning, or dysexecutive states, are found coincident with damage to the frontal lobes. The prefrontal cortex has been implicated in switching set [25] and in several current models, the basal ganglia interface detects patterns of cortical inputs critical to many features of executive functioning [26–30]. These findings implicate the entire fronto-striatal loop with consequences for individuals with Parkinson's disease, vascular dementia, frontotemporal dementia, and even Alzheimer's patients later in the disease.

Evaluation of executive functioning not only has important diagnostic utility but also ramifications for everyday functioning that are important for the clinician to be aware of. For example, deficits in executive functioning correlate with decreased ability to manage medication, pay bills, and cook in patients with even mild AD [31]. These deficits in executive functioning may be subtle and not apparent to the casual observer but have real impact on independence and safety.

Behavior

Behavioral changes occur frequently in dementia and can be at least as disruptive as the cognitive changes. Agitation, aggression, anxiety, disinhibition, delusions/hallucinations, apathy, depression, irritability, and changes in personality and empathy occur with frequency in dementia syndromes [32]. Recognition of behavioral changes in dementia has resulted in the need for increased use of scales measuring neurobehavior [33]. Depression and apathy are described in greater detail later, because distinction between the two is important for diagnostic clarity and the two behaviors are often confused.

Depression

Depression involves both neurovegetative signs and mood changes. The neurovegetative signs can include hypersomnia or insomnia, decreased or increased appetite, decreased energy, weight loss and psychomotor agitation or slowing. Mood changes include depressed mood and feelings of worthlessness, hopelessness, and suicidal ideation. Healthy older adults and demented individuals often experience the vegetative signs of depression but may not experience the pure mood changes. As a result, recognition and diagnosis of depression can be delayed.

Furthermore, depression alone has deleterious effects on cognition. These include decreased concentration and decreased performance on tasks that require significant effort. Therefore, cognitive testing reveals a discrepancy between performance on tests that are effortful versus tests with more automatic responses. Depressed individuals have disproportionate difficulty with memory recall versus recognition [34]. The cognitive difficulties accompanying depression can be quite significant, mimic dementia, and can be difficult to differentiate in routine clinical examination. Differential diagnosis is critical, because treating depression results in amelioration of the cognitive difficulties. As mentioned earlier, having dementia does not preclude depression, but the combination of the two results in excess cognitive disability if the depression is untreated.

Apathy

Apathy is defined as loss of motivation to engage in goal-directed behaviors. From a behavioral perspective, it presents as lack of motivation, decreased initiation, and poor ability to sustain effort. Apathy does not include depressed mood. Apathy and depression share poor motivation and are often confused particularly by caregivers. However, despite similarities apathy is recognized as a separate construct from depression; apathy and depression do not correlate in Parkinson's disease and other neurodegenerative diseases [35–39]. In terms of pathology, apathy is related to disruption of the frontal-basal ganglia circuitry [35,40] and as a result is a significant feature of dementias involving disruption in these brain regions.

Dementia syndromes and neuropsychologic profiles

Mild cognitive impairment

Mild cognitive impairment (MCI) is a diagnosis generally applied to elderly adults who complain of and demonstrate cognitive deficits (predominantly memory) that are beyond typical for normal aging but are not of the severity or quality sufficient for a diagnosis of dementia. The utility of the MCI diagnosis is evidenced by consistent estimates that individuals with MCI are at greater risk for conversion to AD. Despite several methods for operationalizing MCI, the diagnosis is generally applied to individuals with a primary complaint and demonstration of memory difficulties, relative preservation of activities of daily living, and mild to absent changes in other aspects of cognition. Debate continues regarding the most useful way to operationalize the MCI diagnosis. Most MCI classification systems require a subjective memory complaint, informant (eg, family, caretaker) corroboration of memory difficulty, relatively intact activities of daily living, and normal or mild difficulties in nonmemory aspects of cognition. More stringent systems also specify a cutoff point for the severity of memory impairment on standardized neuropsychologic tests (eg, performance < 1.5 SD below the mean) [41]. The rate of MCI conversion to AD is higher than in the general population. Estimates vary, but individuals with MCI progress to AD at a rate of 10% to 25% per year as contrasted with healthy elderly controls who progress at a rate of 1% to 2% per year [42].

Individuals with MCI consistently demonstrate impaired memory [43]. This in part is a reflection of diagnostic criteria such that individuals with mild impairment in other cognitive areas may be missed. The pattern of memory decline found in MCI appears to be degradation of information in memory storage [43]. The storage deficit is seen in the loss of information over time with no improvement in performance when using recognition formats. This pattern of decline is consistent with that found in AD and thought to be evidence that MCI is a preclinical stage of AD.

Recent research reveals early changes in executive functioning, including increased levels of apathy. Individuals with MCI have been found to have impairments in financial management, including difficulties with cash management and bill payment [44]. Given their generally high level of functioning, individuals with these difficulties could go undetected thereby making them vulnerable. Taken together, changes in memory and executive functioning improve prediction of conversion from MCI to AD [43,45].

Alzheimer's disease

AD is the most common form of dementia, accounting for an estimated two thirds of dementia in people 65 years of age or older [46]. Age is the most important risk factor for AD. Other potential risk factors include possession of an APOE Σ4 allele, a family history of AD, low education, female gender, and depression.

Depletion of neurons in the basal forebrain cholinergic system and subsequent loss of acetylcholine correspond with predominant memory deficits. Pathologic diagnosis is made from the presence of amyloid plaques and neurofibrillary tangles. The number of neurofibrillary tangles, neuronal loss, and cognitive dysfunction are correlated in AD [47]. Memory decline is the hallmark of cognitive change in AD. The memory decline in AD is characterized as a storage deficit with rapid forgetting and poor delayed memory [48,49]. As expected, a meta-analysis of cognitive decline in AD reveals that memory is the most severely affected cognitive domain [50]. Individuals with AD tend to confabulate and create answers or responses to questions that are inaccurate [51,52]. Furthermore, on tests of word recall, AD patients have more intrusions of incorrect words and inaccurately recognized words as being on the list (false positives) than individuals with other dementias. Generally, recent memory is affected first, and memory for remote events worsens later in the disease.

Orientation to time and date are disrupted early in the disease, because these abilities require good learning and recent memory. As the disease progresses, orientation worsens to include problems identifying familiar places and family members or other people well known to the individual. In general, deficits in declarative memory are mild initially and progress into severe deficits.

As the disease worsens, procedural memory may decline, and individuals will have difficulty with activities of daily living, including dressing and using utensils. These difficulties can also be characterized as an ideomotor apraxia. On testing, this is often seen when the patient uses a finger as a toothbrush rather than pantomiming holding the toothbrush as asked.

The language difficulties commonly found in AD are consistent with difficulties with semantic memory. AD patients often have problems with word finding, in particular nouns, and coming up with names of people. It is important to take into account that the ability to recall names of people declines with healthy aging, is a common complaint among healthy older individuals, and in and of itself is not a marker for AD. Category fluency (eg, naming animals or furniture) is more impaired than semantic fluency (eg, naming words that begin with a particular letter) perhaps because category fluency is dependent on access to temporal-lobe semantic stores [53,54]. Within category fluency tasks, AD patients have less difficulty naming nonbiologic items, such as clothing or modes of transportation, than biologic items, such as animals or flowers. This relative difficulty increases with dementia severity [55]. As the disease progresses, language difficulties become more pervasive and spoken language may become less meaningful with an increase in comprehension difficulties.

Although deficits in executive functioning exist in AD, they typically are not a prominent feature of the disease, and early in the disease are referable to an underlying deficit in semantic memory and mesial temporal lobe damage [56,57]. However, to the extent that a dysexecutive state exists, the consequences for functional capacity are measurable [31,44].

Behavioral changes in AD include depression, anxiety, and apathy. Depression is present in up to 50% of patients with AD [58]. Depression rates vary by severity and disease stage. Early in the disease, depression may be attributed to awareness of the cognitive changes. Many AD patients experience the neurovegetative signs of depression unrelated to depression—therefore, neurovegetative signs alone are not helpful in differential diagnosis. Furthermore, apathy is often confused with depression, particularly by caregivers, which may help to explain the greater report of depression in patients by caregivers than by patients themselves. In fact, even moderately demented AD patients can reliably report mood states [59]. Apathy is associated with significant caregiver distress and greater use of health care facilities in AD [60]. Apathy is not correlated with dysphoria in AD but is related to executive dysfunction [61].

Vascular dementia

Dementia associated with cerebrovascular disease is second in frequency to AD [62]. The clinical presentation of cognitive changes associated with vascular dementia (VaD) varies according to the cause of cerebral damage. For the most part, large vessel disease leads to cortical infarcts with a cortical presentation. Small vessel disease, often resulting from hypertension, diabetes, or white matter disease, presents with a subcortical picture [63,64]. Relative to AD, the onset is more likely to be sudden and the progression stepwise.

The most prominent cognitive difference between AD and VaD is the relatively spared memory and impaired executive function in the latter group. Unaided recall, recall with cues, and recognition memory are better in VaD than AD [56]. People with VaD may be seen as "forgetful." In fact, recognition memory can be normal in VaD, and the use of recognition cues can greatly enhance independence.

VaD is associated with a dysexecutive state, related to disruption of frontal-subcortical connections, which significantly affects everyday functioning [65]. Patients with VaD have difficulty maintaining "mental set," which translates into difficulty completing tasks. They also have difficulty understanding the nature of novel tasks and inhibiting predicted responses when an alternate response would be more appropriate. On a functional level, these deficits result in slowed thinking, poor problem solving, and limited ability to focus.

Naming is relatively better in VaD than in AD, with VaD patients less likely to make intrusion errors on confrontation naming [66]. Semantic aspects of language are generally intact; however, verbal fluency may be decreased. Visuospatial deficits include difficulties with clock drawing and clock reading, normally a highly familiar task [67].

Behavior and personality changes are a significant component of vascular dementia. Consistent with other frontal-subcortical changes, apathy is common in VaD, is unrelated to overall dementia severity, and accounts for more variance in ability to do basic activities of daily living (ADLs) than does dementia severity [68,69]. Apathy is more common in VaD than in AD [70]. Depression is also a feature of VaD and causes excess disability if left untreated.

Frontotemporal dementias

The three frontotemporal dementia (FTD) subtypes (frontotemporal demential, progressive nonfluent aphasia, and semantic dementia) typically have a younger age of onset than does AD. Prominent behavioral changes occur early in the disease and typically are noticed more than early cognitive changes. FTD patients are distinguishable from AD patients both cognitively and behaviorally [71]. Common behavioral changes include apathy, disinhibition, tactlessness, loss of social graces, and emotional blunting [72,73]. Other changes include a decline in personal hygiene and lack of spontaneity. These changes are usually of greater concern to family members than to patients. Memory and calculation initially are relatively preserved in the FTDs. Attention, abstraction, and reasoning are impaired in these individuals. In general, FTD patients perform poorly on tests of executive functioning.

In progressive nonfluent aphasia, nonfluent speech with stuttering, impaired repetition, and writing changes are followed by late mutism. The ability to produce words by category is relatively better than word production by letter. These patients have relatively preserved social skills early in the disease [74]. In semantic dementia, speech is fluent but empty of meaning with loss of comprehension. Naming, reading, and comprehension are impaired, although patients may be unaware of comprehension difficulties. Naming by letter is relatively better than by category. Other supportive features of semantic dementia include preserved math skills and preoccupation with money. In the frontal variant of FTD, lack of motivation, distractibility, and impaired judgment are common. The frontal variant differs from the other FTDS in that language is relatively preserved.

Parkinson's dementia

Dementia that occurs secondary to Parkinson's dementia (PD) is often unrecognized, but substantial research indicates that significant cognitive changes occur with frequency [75–77]. PD is characterized as a dysexecutive state that involves disruption of the fronto-striatal loop. This results in difficulties with problem solving, abstract thinking, judgment, and slowed processing [77]. Changes in procedural memory are common in PD. Declarative memory changes appear to be due to a retrieval deficit rather than an encoding problem. Cognitive changes can occur early in the disease and have implications for adaptive functioning. Apathy is common and appears to be disease related rather than a reaction to disability [78]. Depression is also a significant but distinct behavioral complication that can exacerbate cognitive functioning [79].

Dementia with Lewy bodies

Dementia with Lewy bodies (DLB) is the most common of the several of the dementias with Parkinsonian features. Diagnostic criteria for DLB include fluctuating cognition, visual hallucinations, and Parkinsonism, including falls and syncope that cannot predate the cognitive decline by more than 1 year. Fluctuating cognition is difficult to operationalize but is frequently reported by caregivers. Fluctuations are reported to take place over several days or less than half an hour. Caregivers may report swings ranging from "normal" cognition to disorientation and confusion. Visual hallucinations are stereotypical and often involve small people, children, or animals. They are rarely experienced as threatening. The cognitive changes in DLB are consistent with fronto-striatal disruption, resulting in diminished executive functioning. Visuoperceptual difficulties, common in DLB, are exacerbated by frequent hallucinations [80].

Summary

Distinct cognitive and behavioral profiles are associated with the different dementias. These profiles fall generally into deficits associated with medial temporal lobe functioning or frontally mediated circuits. Awareness is increasing of dementias involving deficits in frontally mediated circuits. Understanding cognitive profiles can help clinicians with diagnosis, prediction of patterns of decline, and therapeutic options. Clinicians may also use this information to educate caregivers, resulting in improved care and decreased anxiety and caregiver burden.

References

[1] American Psychiatric Association. Diagnostic and statistical manual of mental disorders. 4th edition. Washington, DC: American Psychiatric Association; 1994.

[2] The American Academy of Neurology. International classification of diseases-9 CM for neurologists. 2002 edition. St. Paul MN: The American Academy of Neurology; 2001.

[3] Lezak MD. Neuropsychological assessment. 3rd edition. New York: Oxford University Press, Inc.; 1995.

[4] Folstein MF, Folstein SE, McHugh PR. Mini Mental State. J Psychiatr Res 1975;12:189–98.

[5] Cossa FM, Della Sala S, Musicco M, Spinnler H, Ubezio MC. Comparison of two scoring systems of the Mini-Mental State Examination as a screening test for dementia. J Clin Epidemiol 1997;50(8):961–5.

[6] Norman LA, Borson AJ. An alphabetical "WORLD": a new version of an old test. Neurology 1997;49(6):1521–4.

[7] Miskin M, Appenzeller T. The anatomy of memory. Sci Am 1987;256:80–9.

[8] Squire LR, Zola-Morgan S. The neuropsychology of memory: new links between humans and experimental animals. Annals of the New York Academy of Sciences 1985;444:137–49.

[9] Squire LR. Memory and brain. New York: Oxford University Press; 1987.

[10] Squire LR. Memory and the hippocampus: a synthesis from findings with rats, monkeys, and humans. Psychol Rev 1992;99:195–231.

[11] Bailey CH, Kandel ER. Molecular approaches to the study of short-term and long-term memory. In: Cohen CW, editor. Functions of the brain. Oxford: Clarendon Press; 1985. p. 98–129.

[12] Willingham DB. A neuropsychological theory of motor skill learning. Psychol Rev 1998; 105:558–94.

[13] De Guise E, Del Pesce M, Foschi N, Quattrini A, Papo I, Lassonde M. Callosal and cortical contribution to procedural learning. Brain 1999;122:1049–62.

[14] Robertson EM, Tormos JM, Maeda F, Pascual-Leone A. The role of the dorsolateral prefrontal cortex during sequence learning is specific for spatial information. Cereb Cortex 2001;11(7): 628–35.

[15] Sarazin M, Deweer B, Merkl A, Von Poser N, Pillon B, Dubois B. Procedural learning and striatofrontal dysfunction in Parkinson's disease. Mov Disord 2002;17(2):265–73.

[16] Schmidtke K, Manner H, Kaufmann R, Schmolck H. Cognitive procedural learning in patients with fronto-striatal lesions. Learn Mem 2002;9(6):419–29.

[17] Gazzaniga MS. Perceptual and attentional processes following callosal section in humans. Neuropsychologia 1987;25:119–33.

[18] Hasher L, Zacks RT. Automatic and effortful processes in memory. J Exp Psychol Gen 1979; 108:356–88.

[19] Jemel B, Oades RD, Oknina L, Achenbach C, Ropcke B. Frontal and temporal lobe sources for a marker of controlled auditory attention: the negative difference (Nd) event-related potential. Brain Topogr 2003;15(4):249–62.

[20] Manly T, Owen A, McAvinue L, Datta A, Lewis G, Scott S, et al. Enhancing the sensitivity of a sustained attention task to frontal damage: convergent clinical and functional imaging evidence. Neurocase 2003;9(4):340–9.
[21] West R. Neural correlates of cognitive control and conflict detection in the Stroop and digit-location tasks. Neuropsychologia 2003;41:1122–35.
[22] Gazzaniga MS, Ivry RB, Mangun GR. Cognitive neuroscience, the biology of the mind. 2nd edition. New York: WW Norton and Company, Inc.; 2002.
[23] Haaland KY, Harrington MF, Knight RT. Spatial deficits in ideomotor limb apraxia. A kinematic analysis of aiming movements. Brain 1999;122:1169–82.
[24] Benson DF. Classical syndromes of aphasia. In: Boller F, Grafman J, editors. Handbook of neuropsychology, vol. 1. Amsterdam: Elsevier; 1988. p. 267–80.
[25] Otani S. Memory trace in prefrontal cortex: theory for the cognitive switch. Biol Rev Camb Philos Soc 2002;77(4):563–77.
[26] Redgrave P, Prescott TJ, Gurney K. The basal ganglia: a vertebrate solution to the selection problem? Neuroscience 1999;89:1009–23.
[27] Kropotov JD, Etlinger S. Selection of actions in the basal ganglia-thalamocortical circuits: review and model. Int J Psychophysiol 1999;31:197–217.
[28] Mink J. The basal ganglia: focused selection and inhibition of competing motor programs. Prog Neurobiol 1996;50:381–425.
[29] Houghton G, Tipper SP. Inhibitory mechanisms of neural and cognitive control: applications to selective attention and sequential action. Brain and Cognition 1996;30(1):20–43.
[30] Hikosaka O. Neural systems for control of voluntary action-a hypothesis. Adv Biophys 1998; 35:81.
[31] Boyle PA, Malloy PF, Salloway S, Cahn-Weiner DA, Coben R, Cummings J. Evecutive dysfunction and apathy predict functional impairment in Alzheimer disease. Am J Geriatr Psychiatry 2003;11(2):214–21.
[32] Cummings JL. Frontal-subcortical circuits and human behavior. Arch Neurol 1993;50:873–80.
[33] Miller BL, Diehl J, Freedman M, Kertesz A, Mendez M, Rascovsky K. International approaches to frontotemporal dementia diagnosis: from social cognition to neuropsychology. Ann Neurol 2003;54(5):S7–10.
[34] Ilsley JE, Moffoot AP, O'Carroll RE. An analysis of memory dysfunction in major depression. J Affect Disord 1995;35(1–2):1–9.
[35] Aarsland D, Larsen JP, Lim NG, Janvin C, Karlsen K, Tandberg E, et al. Range of neuropsychiatric disturbances in patients with Parkinson's disease. J Neurol Neurosurg Psychiatry 1999;67:492–6.
[36] Assal F, Cummings JL. Neuropsychiatric symptoms in the dementias. Curr Opin Neurol 2002; 15:445–50.
[37] Levy ML, Cummings JL, Fairbanks LA, Masterman D, Miller BL, Craig AH, et al. Apathy is not depression. J Neuropsychiatry Clin Neurosci 1998;10:314–9.
[38] Pluck GC, Brown RG. Apathy in Parkinson's disease. J Neurol Neurosurg Psychiatry 2002; 73:636–42.
[39] Strauss ME, Sperry SD. An informant-based assessment of apathy in Alzheimer disease. Neuropsychiatry Neuropsychol Behav Neurol 2002;15(3):176–83.
[40] Isella V, Melzi P, Grimaldi M, Iurlaro S, Piolti R, Ferrarese C, et al. Clinical, neuropsychological, and morphometric correlates of apathy in Parkinson's disease. Mov Disord 2002;17:366–71.
[41] Petersen RC. Aging, mild cognitive impairment, and Alzheimer's disease. Neurol Clin 2000; 18(4):789–806.
[42] Petersen RC, Stevens JC, Ganguli M, Tangalos EG, Cummings JL, DeKosky ST. Practice parameter: early detection of dementia: mild cognitive impairment (an evidence-based review). Neurology 2001;56:1133–42.
[43] Crowell TA, Luis CA, Vanderploeg RD, Schinka JA, Mullan M. Memory patterns and executive functioning in mild cognitive impairment and Alzheimer's disease. Aging Neuropsychol Cogn 2002;9(4):288–97.

[44] Griffith HR, Belue K, Sicola A, Krzywanski S, Zamrini E, Harrell L, et al. Impaired financial abilities in mild cognitive impairment: a direct assessment approach. Neurology 2003;60:449–57.
[45] Ready RE, Ott BR, Grace J, Cahn-Weiner DA. Apathy and executive dysfunction in mild cognitive impairment and Alzheimer disease. Am Geriatr Psychiatry 2003;11(2):222–8.
[46] Geldmacher DS. Contemporary diagnosis and management of Alzheimer's disease. Pennsylvania: Handbooks in Health Care Co., a Division of AMM Co., Inc.; 2003.
[47] Masliah E, Katzman RD. Role of synaptic pathology in the mechanisms of dementia of the Alzheimer's type. Clin Neurosci 1993;1:192–8.
[48] Paulsen JS, Salmon DP, Monsch AU, Butters N, Swenson MR, Bondi MW. Discrimination of cortical from subcortical dementias on the basis of memory and problem-solving tests. J Clin Psychol 1995;51(1):48–58.
[49] Welsh KA, Mirra S, Fillenbaum G, Gearing M, Beekly D, Edland S. Neuropsychological and neuropathological differences of Alzheimer's disease from other dementias: The CERAD experience. Presented at the 24th annual meeting of the International Neuropsychological Society. Chicago, February 14–17, 1996.
[50] Christensen H, Hadzi-Pavlovic D, Jacomb P. The psychometric differentiation of dementia in normal aging: a meta-analysis. Psychol Assess 1991;3:147–55.
[51] Kern RS, Van Gorp WG, Cummings JL, Brown WS, Osato SS. Confabulation in Alzheimer's disease. Brain Cogn 1992;19(2):172–82.
[52] Tallberg IM, Almkvist O. Confabulation and memory in patients with Alzheimer's disease. J Clin Exp Neuropsychol 2001;23(2):172–84.
[53] Cerhan JH, Ivnik RJ, Smith GE, Tangalos EC, Petersen RC, Boeve BF. Diagnostic utility of letter fluency, category fluency, and fluency difference scores in Alzheimer's disease. Clin Neuropsychol 2002;16(1):35–42.
[54] Vliet EC, Manly J, Tang MX, Marder K, Bell K, Stern Y. The neuropsychological profiles of mild Alzheimer's disease and questionable dementia as compared to age-related cognitive decline. J Int Neuropsychol Soc 2003;9(5):720–32.
[55] Whatmough C, Chertkow H, Murtha S, Hanratty K. Dissociable brain regions process object meaning and object structure during picture naming. Neuropsychologia 2002;40(2):174–86.
[56] Traykov L, Baudie S, Thibaudet MC, Rigaud AS, Smagghe A, Boller F. Neuropsychological deficit in early subcortical vascular dementia comparison to Alzheimer's disease. Dement Geriatr Cogn Disord 2002;14(1):26–32.
[57] Rascovsky K, Salmon DP, Ho GJ, Galasko D, Peavy GM, Hansen LA, et al. Cognitive profiles differ in autopsy-confirmed frontotemporal dementia and AD. Neurology 2002;58(12):1801–8.
[58] Lyketsos CG, Steele C, Baker L, et al. Major and minor depression in Alzheimer's disease: prevalence and impact. J Neuropsychiatry Clin Neurosci 1997;9:556–61.
[59] Katz IR. Diagnosis and treatment of depression in patients with Alzheimer's disease and other dementias. J Clin Psychiatry 1998;59:38–44.
[60] Clyburn LD, Stones MJ, Hadjistavropoulos T, et al. Predicting caregiver burden and depression in Alzheimer's disease. J Gerentol Behav Psychol Sci Soc 2000;55:S2–13.
[61] McPherson S, Fairbanks L, Tiken S, Cummings JL, Back-Madruga C. Apathy and executive function in Alzheimer's disease. J Int Neuropsychol Soc 2002;8:373–81.
[62] O'Brien JT, Erkinjuntti T, Reisberg B, Roman G, Sawada T, Pantoni L, et al. Vascular cognitive impairment. Lancet Neurol 2003;2:89–98.
[63] Roman GC. Defining dementia: clinical criteria for the diagnosis of vascular dementia. Acta Neurol Scand 2002;106(Suppl 178):6–9.
[64] Roman GC. Vascular dementia: distinguishing characteristics, treatment and prevention. J Am Geriatr Soc 2003;51:S296–304.
[65] Cannata AP, Alberoni M, Franceschi M, Mariani C. Frontal impairment in subcortical ischemic vascular dementia in comparison to Alzheimer's disease. Dement Geriatr Cogn Disord 2002; 13:101–11.
[66] Huff FJ. Language in normal aging and age-related neurological diseases. In: Boller F, Grafman J, editors. Handbook of neuropsychology, vol.4. Elsevier: Amsterdam; 1990. p. 251–64.

[67] Schmidtke K, Hull M. Neuropsychological differentiation of small vessel disease, Alzheimer's disease and mixed dementia. J Neurol Sci 2002;(203–4):17–22.

[68] Ahron-Peretz J, Kliot D, Tomer R. Behavioral differences between white matter lacunar dementia and Alzheimer's disease: a comparison on the neuropsychiatric inventory. Dement Geriatr Cogn Disord 2000;11(5):294–8.

[69] Zawacki TW, Grace J, Paul R, Moser DJ, Ott BR, Gordon N, et al. Behavioral problems as predictors of functional abilities of vascular dementia patients. J Neuropsychiatry Clin Neurosci 2002;14:296–302.

[70] Hargrave R, Geck LC, Reed B, Mungas D. Affective behavioural disturbances in Alzheimer's disease and ischemic vascular disease. J Neurol Neurosurg Psychiatry 2000;68:41–6.

[71] Moretti R, Torre P, Antonello RM, Cazzato G. Fronto-temporal dementia versus Alzheimer disease. Arch Gerentol Geriatr 2001;33(Suppl 1):273–8.

[72] Boone KB, Miller BL, Swartz R, Lu P, Lee A. Relationship between positive and negative symptoms and neuropsychological scores in frontotemporal dementia and Alzheimer's disease. J Int Neuropsychol Soc 2003;9:698–709.

[73] Snowden JS, Gibbons ZC, Blackshaw A, Doubleday E, Thompson J, Craufurd D, et al. Social cognition in frontotemporal dementia and Huntington's disease. Neuropsychologia 2003;41: 688–701.

[74] Nestor P, Hodges J. Non-Alzheimer dementias. Semin Neurol 2000;20(4):439–46.

[75] Levy G, Jacobs DM, Tang MX, Cote LJ, Louis ED, Alfaro B, et al. Memory and executive function impairment predict dementia in Parkinson's disease. Mov Disord 2002;17(6):1221–6.

[76] Lewis S, Dove A, Robbins TW, Barker RA, Owen AM. Cognitive impairments in early Parkinson's disease are accompanied by reductions in activity in frontostriatal neural circuitry. J Neurosci 2003;23(15):6351–6.

[77] Saint-Cyr JA. Neuropsychology for movement disorders neurosurgery. Can J Neurol Sci 2003; 30(1):S83–93.

[78] Pluck GC, Brown RG. Apathy in Parkinson's disease. J Neurol Neurosurg Psychiatry 2002;73: 636–42.

[79] Uekermann J, Daum I, Peters S, Wiebel B, Przuntek H, Muller T. Depressed mood and executive dysfunction in early Parkinson's disease. Acta Neurol Scand 2003;107:341–8.

[80] Simard M, van Reekum R, Myran D. Visuospatial impairment in dementia with Lewy bodies and Alzheimer's disease: a process analysis approach. Int J Geriatr Psychiatry 2003;18(5):387–91.

ELSEVIER
SAUNDERS

Clin Geriatr Med 20 (2004) 59–68

CLINICS IN GERIATRIC MEDICINE

Cholinesterase inhibitors in the treatment of Alzheimer's disease and related dementias

Donna Masterman, MD[a,b,*]

[a]*Department of Neurology, David Geffen School of Medicine at UCLA, 710 Westwood Plaza, Box 951769, Los Angeles, CA 90095-1769, USA*
[b]*Amgen, Inc., 1 Amgen Center Drive, MS 38-3-A, Thousand Oaks, CA 91320, USA*

Alzheimer's disease (AD) is the most common cause of dementia in the elderly and afflicts an estimated 2 to 4 million people in the United States [1], a number that can be projected to increase to 14 million by the year 2050. It accounts for 40% to 59% of nursing home admissions [2] and imposes an expanding economic burden on patients, their families, and the nation. It is the third most expensive disease to treat in the United States behind heart disease and cancer with an overall estimated annual cost between $80 and $100 billion. Effective treatments are urgently needed. Symptomatic treatments can help delay nursing home placement and thereby reduce costs substantially as well as provide relevant benefit to patients and their families. This article provides a brief overview of the current use of cholinesterase inhibitors in the treatment of AD with a look toward new potential uses in AD and related dementias.

Review of acetylcholinesterase inhibitors

Acetylcholinesterase inhibitors (AChEIs) have been approved by the US Food & Drug Administration (FDA) for the symptomatic treatment of AD since 1993 beginning with tacrine hydrochloride, followed by the introduction of donepezil hydrochloride in 1997, rivastigmine tartrate in 2000, and galantamine hydrobromide in 2001. Use of these drugs has become accepted as the standard of care in the treatment of mild to moderate AD. The basis for their use is predicated on the cholinergic hypothesis. Selective loss of cholinergic neurons is known to occur in AD, resulting in a profound reduction in the levels of the neurotransmitter acetylcholine, an important transmitter in learning and memory neuronal circuitry. The four currently approved AChEIs have all been demonstrated

* Amgen, Inc., 1 Amgen Center Drive, MS 38-3-A, Thousand Oaks, CA 91320.
E-mail address: donnam@amgen.com

doi:10.1016/j.cger.2003.11.002

to have clear efficacy on cognition, and most also showed a benefit in day-to-day function and behavioral symptoms in patients with mild to moderate disease. Longer range follow-up studies now point to AChEIs having not only a symptomatic effect but also a stabilizing effect, suggesting a potential disease-modifying influence. The role of these compounds on AD pathogenesis is unclear, but emerging data suggest an interaction of AChEIs with amyloid processing in the brain [3–7].

Pharmacokinetics

Tacrine (tetrahydroaminoacridine) was the first AChEI approved by the FDA for the symptomatic treatment of mild to moderate AD, but it has been primarily replaced by the newer generation AChEIs that have a more favorable side effect profile and dosing regimen.

Donepezil hydrochloride was the first of a newer class of reversible AChEIs. It is a piperidine and does not contain the acridine group that had been linked to the heptatoxicity and has specificity for the neuronal form of AChE with little butyrlcholinesterase (BChE) inhibition. It is metabolized by the P450 enzyme system and eliminated via the liver. The long half-life allows for once daily dosing, and although it is recommended to titrate up to the highest dose of 10 mg after 4 to 6 weeks, the starting dose of 5 mg is also effective.

Rivastigmine tartrate is a carbamate acetylcholinesterase inhibitor with selectivity for the central nervous system. It is pseudo-irreversible, meaning the drug has a prolonged duration of action with AChE being inhibited for several hours after the drug has been metabolized and eliminated [8]. Drug metabolism does not use the hepatic cytochrome P450 enzyme system. The starting dose is 1.5 mg twice a day, which is then to be titrated up to 3.0 twice a day after 2 or more weeks, and finally aiming for a dose of 6 mg twice a day. The drug is generally well tolerated with the principle side effect being gastrointestinal, which is often transient and is aided by taking the medication on a full stomach.

Galantamine is a phenanthrene alkaloid isolated from the European daffodil or common snowdrop and is a reversible inhibitor of AChE [9]. It is also a modulator of nicotinic acetylcholine receptors in the brain. It is metabolized by the cytochrome P450 enzyme system and yields a potent metabolite, sanguinine, which is three times as powerful as the parent compound and accounts for 20% of the administered galantamine. No liver toxicity has been reported, but as with the other AChEIs, gastrointestinal symptoms are the most common side effect and occur in $< 4\%$ of patients on galantamine [10]. It has a half-life of 5 to 7 hours and is dosed twice a day beginning with a starting dose of 4 mg and titrating up every 4 weeks to 8 mg or 12 mg twice a day.

Table 1 provides a summary of the pharmacokinetics for each of the most commonly used AChEIs. All of these drugs have been shown in clinical trials to be safe and generally well tolerated, with gastrointestinal symptoms as the most common side effect. In clinical trials, gastrointestinal side effects were greatest with rivastigmine, least common with donepezil, and intermediate with

Table 1
Acetylcholinesterase inhibitor pharmacokinetic characteristics

Drug	Donepezil	Rivastigmine	Galantamine
Trade name	Aricept[a]	Exelon[b]	Reminyl[c]
Drug class	Piperidine	Carbamate	Alkaloid
AChEI / BChEI	+++	+	+
Reversibility	Reversible	Pseudo-irreversible	Reversible
Elimination	Hepatic	Renal	Renal + Hepatic
Metabolism	CYP2D6 and CYP3A4	AChE-mediated hydrolysis	CYP2D6 and CYP3A4
Protein binding	96%	40%	18%
$T_{1/2}$	70–80 hours	2 hours	5–7 hours
Effective dose	5–10 mg/day	6–12 mg/day	16–24 mg/day
Dosing frequency	qd	bid	bid

[a] Eisai, Teaneck, New Jersey.
[b] Novartis, East Hanover, New Jersey.
[c] Janssen Pharmaceutica, Titusville, New Jersey.

galantamine. Other potential side effects of AChEIs included syncope, muscle cramps, sleep disturbance, behavioral agitation, and urinary incontinence.

Efficacy of acetylcholinesterase inhibitors in mild to moderate Alzheimer's disease

Cognitive improvement in patients with mild to moderate AD has been demonstrated for each of the approved AChEIs in several large, multi-centered, double-blind, randomized, placebo-controlled clinical trials [8,11–17]. The treatment benefit on the Alzheimer's Disease Assessment Scale-cognitive subscale or ADAS-cog (the standard instrument used to measure cognitive function in AD clinical trials) has typically been shown in short-term 6-month placebo-controlled trials. A 12-month double-blind, placebo-controlled trial using donepezil has been conducted showing continued efficacy compared with controls at 1 year [18]. Longer term open-label trials have also been conducted with donepezil, rivastigmine, and galantamine—each demonstrating a slowing or stabilization effect when compared with historical controls (Table 2).

In addition to extended open-label clinical trial data out to 3 years suggesting clinical benefit over the expected natural history of decline, other relevant long-

Table 2
Prospective studies evaluating the long-term treatment effects of AChEIs in AD

Study	AChEI	Number randomized	Treatment duration (years)
Winblad et al 2001 [18]	Donepezil	286	1
Raskind et al 2000 [12]	Galantamine	636	1
Rogers and Friedhoff 1996 [15]	Donepezil	1500	2
Mohs et al 2001 [19]	Donepezil	431	2
Anand et al 1998 [8]	Rivastigmine	2149	2
Doody et al 2001 [20]	Donepezil	763	2.8
Rainer and Mucke 1999 [21]	Galantamine	44	3

term outcome data extend to the impact of AChEIs on rate of nursing home placement. In a retrospective, open-label study of AD patients followed for 8 years who were enrolled in a memory clinic and treated with AChEIs (96% were on donepezil), a highly significant difference was found in the risk for placement in a nursing home compared with a group of dementia patients who were matched for characteristics and co-morbid conditions [22]. In another study, persistent exposure to donepezil 5 or 10 mg/day in the context initially of a clinical trial with extended follow-up was associated with a 21.4-month mean delay in nursing home placement when compared with a group of patients with minimal donepezil exposure [23].

Acetylcholinesterase inhibitors in moderate to severe Alzheimer's disease

The approval of the currently available AChEIs was based on their efficacy and safety data in patients with mild to moderate disease, but subsequent studies suggest that they may also be of benefit in more advanced stages of the illness. Feldman and colleagues [24] reported on the results of a 24-week, multi-centered, randomized, double-blind, placebo-controlled clinical trial involving patients with moderate to severe AD. This study involved 290 subjects with Mini-Mental State Exam (MMSE) scores ranging from 5 to 17 and found significant improvement in subjects treated with donepezil compared with placebo in the primary outcome measure, the Clinician's Interview-Based Impression of Change with caregiver input (CIBIC +) as well as cognitive function, behavior, and activities of daily living. The cognitive measure used in this study was the Severe Impairment Battery (SIB). The mean decline on the SIB in placebo subjects was roughly 3 points during the 24-week study. By contrast there was improvement in the donepezil-treated group of a similar magnitude. The mean treatment difference was about 6 points. There was no change on the MMSE [25] during the 24 weeks for the placebo group, while there was a 1.5-point improvement on the donepezi-treated group. Significant improvements were also found in measures of activities of daily living and behavioral symptoms. The behavioral symptoms as measured by the Neuropsychiatric Inventory (NPI) [26] improved from baseline with donepezil by 4.6 points. Individual item analysis at week 24 showed a significant difference in depression/dysphoria, anxiety, and apathy.

Rivastigmine has also been reported to benefit the behavioral symptoms in a multi-center study of open-label rivastigmine in 173 AD patients residing in nursing homes. Cummings and colleagues [27] found that 58% demonstrated improvement in behavioral problems that included significant responses for irritability, aberrant motor behavior, apathy, hallucinations, disruptive night-time behavior, agitation, and delusions. A post hoc analysis of more moderately advanced AD patients that were part of the pivotal trial was performed, demonstrating benefit in this more advanced patient population as well [28].

Galantamine has also been found in a randomized, double-blind, placebo-controlled clinical trial in outpatients with mild to moderate AD to have a beneficial effect on neuropsychiatric symptoms [17]. The total NPI score was improved in the group of subjects receiving galantamine compared with placebo, and the specific neuropsychiatric symptoms of anxiety, disinhibition, hallucinations, and aberrant motor behavior were significantly improved and the degree of caregiver distress reduced ($P < 0.05$). Wilkinson et al [29] reported the results of a post hoc analysis of a more advanced cohort of AD patients (MMSE 10–12) who participated in the pivotal trials with galantamine revealed a beneficial response in this patient population.

In a recent meta-analysis of the published literature on the effects of AChEI on behavioral symptoms, Trinh and colleagues [17], reviewed the published literature on the topic from 1966 to 2001. They reported on the 29 parallel-group or crossover randomized, double-blind, placebo-controlled trials of outpatients with mild to moderate AD treated for at least 1 month with a AChEI; 16 trials included evaluations of neuropsychiatric symptoms. A small, but statistically significant improvement was seen with AChEI use.

In addition to behavioral symptoms, progressive functional decline is also a major challenge in the later stages of AD; together these symptoms drive caregiver distress and leads to an increased need for in home supportive care or institutionalization. The slower decline in functional loss as activities of daily living in patients with moderately severe disease associated with donepezil resulted in caregivers reporting less time spent assisting with the activities of daily living (ADLs) and in lower levels of caregiver stress [30].

Acetylcholinesterase inhibitors in vascular dementia

Vascular dementia (VaD) is the second most common cause of dementia in the elderly and is a growing public health concern. Of stroke survivors over the age of 65, approximately one third will have VaD. In addition, overlap exists between these two common causes of dementia, AD and VaD, and mixed cases are not uncommon. It is also increasingly recognized that cerebrovascular disease may play an additive role in patients with AD. In addition to emphasizing the importance of addressing vascular risk factors in the management of patients with VaD or AD with cerebrovascular disease, increasing evidence suggests that patients with VaD also exhibit a cholinergic deficit and may be responsive the AChEI therapy. A recent randomized, double blind, placebo-controlled, multicenter, international 24-week study of galantamine in patients with both VaD and mixed VaD + AD was performed in 592 subjects [31]. In this study 49% of the subjects had a mixture of AD + cerebrovascular disease, 42% had VaD based on NINDS-ARIEN criteria, and another 9% had nonspecific missed dementia with neuroimaging evidence of cerebrovascular disease. Overall the galantamine-treated group demonstrated a statistically significant improvement in cognition as measured by the ADAS-cog compared with the placebo treated group ($P = 0.0006$). Even though the study was not designed to detect an effect of galantamine on pure VaD, a trend toward improvement was observed.

In a larger clinical trial with donepezil, 1219 subjects were recruited in a randomized, placebo-controlled, multi-center, multinational study in patients with possible or probable VaD according to NINDS-AIREN criteria for 24 weeks. This study examined a more pure VaD group and found significant improvements over placebo-treated patients in both cognition (ADAS-cog) and on an assessment of global function (CIBIC +) [18,32,33].

A smaller open-label study of rivastigmine in the treatment of VaD was recently reported on in 16 subjects followed for 22 months [34].

Acetylcholinesterase inhibitors in dementia with Lewy bodies

Demential with Lewy bodies (DLB) has been recognized during the last decade and a half as a common form of dementia in the elderly accounting for 15% to 25% of all dementia presentations [35]. Fluctuating cognitive impairment and attention deficits are usually accompanied by recurrent visual hallucinations and Parkinsonism [36]. DLB patients also have profound cholinergic deficits. In an open-label, 6-month study, use of donepezil resulted in substantial improvement of behavioral symptoms and cognition in patients with DLB [37]. A larger, international Lewy body dementia trial was conducted with rivastigmine in a double-blind, placebo-controlled, 20-week clinical study set up to evaluate the safety and efficacy in 120 patients with DLB who were randomized to rivastigmine or placebo [38]. The mean age in both groups was 73.9 years, and the baseline MMSE scores were 17.9 and 17.8, respectively, in the rivastigmine and placebo groups. The primary objectives for this study were to determine the effects of rivastigmine on the core behavioral symptoms using the four-item NPI psychopathology cluster (hallucinations, delusions, depression, and apathy) and to determine the effect of rivastigmine on cognitive deficits using the sum of speed/attention scores from the computerized battery (cognitive drug research [CDR]). These were the symptoms observed most frequently in the DLB patients at baseline [39]. The CDR is a computerized test that assesses cognitive functioning in patients with organic disorders. It evaluates cognitive skills of attention, short-term and long-term memory, and visuomotor functioning [40].

Significant ($P < 0.01$ versus placebo) improvements were noted in behavioral symptoms, particularly apathy, anxiety, delusions, and hallucinations [41]. Marked improvements in attention and memory also were observed, and Parkinsonian features were not adversely affected. Importantly, these effects were sustained for more than 52 weeks. Grace and colleagues [42] reported on a smaller pilot trial of open-label treatment with rivastigmine in 29 DLB patients who were followed for 96 weeks. No detectable declines in cognition as measured by the MMSE or of neuropsychiatric symptoms as measured by the NPI were seen, and scores were no worse than baseline. Also no deterioration in Parkinsonism was seen during the treatment period.

Donepezil has been reported to be beneficial in DLB, although no blinded studies have been reported. Several case series and reports have shown improvement in cognition using the MMSE, with scores increasing by up to four points. Neuropsychiatric improvement, particularly in the area of hallucinations, has been reported following treatment with donepezil [43,44]. Agitation and delirium-like features common in DLB have likewise been shown to improve [45–47]. Donepezil is generally well tolerated in patients with DLB with only 3% of the patients published in the literature discontinuing the drug due to adverse events that were predominantly gastrointestinal. However, worsening of Parkinsonism has been reported as a not uncommon side effect.

Acetylcholinesterase inhibitors in the treatment of Parkinson's disease

Overt dementia may occur in 30% to 40% of Parkinson's disease (PD) patients, and more subtle intellectual impairment is seen in the majority of patients. The dementia in PD might be explained by the co-occurrence of AD in some cases. However, in many cases the cholinergic system is prominently affected in the absence of cortical Alzheimer's pathology. Whitehouse and colleagues [48] demonstrated that there was a profound loss of cholinergic neurons in the nucleus basalis in PD patients with dementia. There have been a few small studies examining the effects of AChEI on the treatment of dementia associated with PD. Donepezil was significantly ($P < 0.05$) better than placebo in improving cognitive performance, with no increase in Parkinsonian symptoms during treatment [2].

At 12 and 26 weeks, rivastigmine significantly improved Alzheimer's Disease Assessment Scale subscores for recognition ($P = 0.007$), remembering instructions ($P = 0.008$), and concentration ($P = 0.005$) in patients with PD-associated dementia [49]. Moreover, Parkinsonian symptoms did not worsen, as assessed by the Unified Parkinson's Disease Rating Scale. According to the Clinical Global Impression of Change, mild to moderate improvement ($P < 0.0001$) was noted by patients, caregivers, and neurologists [49]. In a separate study, patients with PD dementia who received rivastigmine showed significant improvements in NPI subscores for hallucinations and sleep ($P < 0.02$, $P < 0.015$, respectively) [50].

In another recent case series using galantamine in patients with PD dementia, Aarsland and colleagues [51] reported improvements in global mental symptoms in eight of the 16 patients with some worsening in four following 8 weeks of open-label treatment. Hallucinations improved in seven of nine patients who had experienced them before initiation of galantamine, and Parkinsonism improved in six patients with a mild worsening of tremor experienced in three. A similar trial with donepezil in a small series of patients with PD also revealed some benefit [52].

It is clear from these small series that larger, double-blind, placebo-controlled trials of AChEIs in PDD are warranted and are currently underway.

Summary

AChEIs will continue to play an important role in the treatment armamentarium for AD even as newer strategies for treatment are being explored. A combination approach to treatment may be even more beneficial. AchEIs may play an increasingly important role in the treatment of other related dementias such as VaD, DLB, and PD dementia for which dementia-specific therapies do not exist, but further definitive studies are clearly needed. AChEIS may also have a role in the very early manifestations of disease, such as in mild cognitive impairment. Much work is being directed toward these questions, not only with AChEIs but also with other potential disease-modifying strategies. An active search for new drugs that provide symptomatic improvement of cognitive and functional status in AD patients and may also have an impact on the underlying disease process is underway.

References

[1] Evans DA, Funkenstein H, Albert MS, et al. Prevalence of Alzheimer's disease in a community population of older persons: higher than previously reported. JAMA 1989;262:2551–6.
[2] Katzman R, Aronson M, Fuld PA, et al. Development of dementia in an 80-year-old volunteer cohort. Ann Neurol 1989;25:317–24.
[3] Auld DS, Kornecook TJ, Bastianetto S, Quirion R. Alzheimer's disease and the basal forebrain cholinergic system: relations to beta-amyloid peptides, cognition, and treatment strategies. Prog Neurobiol 2002;68:209–45.
[4] Giacoboni E. Do cholinesterase inhibitors have disease-modifying effects in Alzheimer's disease? CNS Drugs 2001;15:85–91.
[5] Mori F, Lai CC, Fusi F, et al. Cholinesterase inhibitors increase secretion of APPs in rat brain cortex. Neuroreport 1995;6:633–6.
[6] Pakaski M, Kasa P. Role of acetylcholinesterase inhibitors in the metabolism of amyloid precursor protein. Curr Drug Target CNS Neurol Disord 2003;2:163–71.
[7] Rees TM, Brimijoin S. The role of acetylcholinesterase in the pathogenesis of Alzheimer's disease. Drugs Today 2003;39:75–83.
[8] Anand R, Gharabawi G, Enz A. Efficacy and safety results of the early phase studies with exelon (ENA-713) in Alzheimer's disease: an overview. J Drug Dev Clin Pract 1998;8:1–14.
[9] Nordberg A, Svensson A-L. Cholinesterase inhibitors in the treatment of Alzheimer's disease. A comparison of tolerability and pharmacology. Drug Saf 1998;19(6):465–80.
[10] Rainer M. Clinical studies of galanthamine. Drugs Today 1997;4:273–9.
[11] Corey-Bloom J, Anand R, Veach J, for the ENA 713 B352 Study Group. A randomized trial evaluating the efficacy and safety of ENA 713 (rivastigmine tartrate), a new acetylcholinesterase inhibitor, in patients with mild to moderately severe Alzheimer's disease. Intl J of Geriatr Psychopharmacol 1998;1:55–65.
[12] Raskind MA, Peskind ER, Wessel T, et al. Galantamine in AD. A 6-month, randomized, placebo-controlled trial with a 6-month extension. Neurology 2000;54:2261–8.
[13] Rogers SL, Farlow MR, Doody RS, et al. A 24-week double blind placebo controlled trial of donepezil in patients with Alzheimer's disease. Neurology 1998;50:136–45.
[14] Rogers SL, Friedhoff LT, and the Donepezil Study Group. The efficacy and safety of donepezil in patients with Alzheimer's disease. Results of a US multicenter randomized double blind placebo controlled trial. Dementia 1996;7:293–303.
[15] Rojas-Fernandez C. Successful use of donepezil for the treatment of dementia with Lewy bodies. Ann Pharmacother 2001;35:202–5.
[16] Samuel W, Caligiuri M, Galasko D, et al. Better cognitive and psychopathologic response to donepezil in patients prospectively diagnosed as dementia with Lewy bodies: a preliminary study. Int J Geriatr Psychiatry 2000;15:794–802.
[17] Trinh NH, Hoblyn J, Mohanty S, Yaffe K. Efficacy of cholinesterase inhibitors in the treatment

of neuropsychiatric symptoms and functional impairment in Alzheimer disease. JAMA 2003; 289:210–6.
[18] Winblad B, Engedal K, Soininen H, et al. A 1-year, randomized, placebo-controlled study of donepezil in patients with mild to moderate AD. Neurology 2001;57:489–95.
[19] Doody RS, Geldmacher DS, Gordon B, et al, for the Donepezil Study Group. Open-label, multicenter, phase 3 extension study of the safety and efficacy of donepezil in patients with Alzheimer's disease. Arch Neurol 2001;58:427–33.
[20] Mohs RC, Doody RS, Morris JC, et al. A 1-year, placebo-controlled preservation of function survival study of donepezil in AD patients. Neurology 2001;57:481–8.
[21] Rainer M, Mucke HAM. Long-term cognitive benefit from galanthamine in alzheimer's disease. Int J Geriatr Psychiatry 1999;1:197–201.
[22] Lopez OL, Becker JT, Wisniewski S, et al. Cholinesterase inhibitor treatment alters the natural history of Alzheimer's disease. J Neurol Neurosurg Psychiatry 2002;72:310–4.
[23] Geldmacher DS, Provenzano G, McRae T, et al. Donepezil is associated with delayed nursing home placement in patients with Alzheimer's disease. J Am Geriatr Soc 2003;51:937–44.
[24] Feldman H, Gauthier S, Hecker J, et al. A 24-week, randomized, double-blind study of donepezil in moderate to severe Alzheimer's disease. Neurology 2001;57:613–20.
[25] Folstein MF, Folstein SE, McHugh PR. "Mini-Mental State" a practical method for grading the cognitive state of patients for the clinician. J Psychiatr Res 1975;12(3):189–98.
[26] Cummings JL, Mega M, Gray K, et al. The neuropsychiatric inventory: comprehensive assessment of psychopathology in dementia. Neurology 1994;44:2308–14.
[27] Cummings JL, Anand R, Koumaras B. Rivastigmine provides behavioral benefits to Alzheimer's disease patients residing in a nursing home: findings from a 26-week trial. Neurology 2000; 54(Suppl 3):A469.
[28] Doraiswamy PM, Krishnan KRR, Anand R, et al. Long-term effects of rivastigmine in moderately severe Alzheimer's disease: does early initiation of therapy offer sustained benefits? Prog Neuropsychopharmacol Biol Psychiatry 2002;26:705–12.
[29] Wilkinson D, Doody R, Helme R, et al. Donepezil in vascular dementia: a randomized, placebo-controlled study. Neurology 2003;61:479–86.
[30] Feldman H, Gauthier S, Hecker J, et al. Efficacy of donepezil on maintenance of activities of daily living in patients with moderate to severe Alzheimer's disease and the effect on caregiver burden. J Am Geriatr Soc 2003;51:737–44.
[31] Erkinjuntti T, Kurz A, Gautheir S, et al. Efficacy of galantamine in probable vascular dementia and Alzheimer's disease combined with cerebrovascular disease: a randomized trial. Lancet 2002;359:1283–90.
[32] Black S, Roman GC, Geldmacher D, et al. Efficacy and tolerability of donepezil in vascular dementia: positive results of a 24-week, multicenter, international, randomized, placebo-controlled clinical trial. Stroke 2003;34(10):2323–30.
[33] Pratt RD, Perdomo CA. Results of clinical studies with donepezil in vascular dementia. Am J Geriatr Psychiatry 2002;10(Suppl 1):88–9.
[34] Moretti R, Torre P, Antonello RM, et al. Rivastigmine in subcortical vascular dementia: an open 22-month study. J Neurol Sci 2002;203–204:141–6.
[35] Perry EK, Haroutunian V, Perry RH, et al. Neocortical cholinergic activities differentiate Lewy body dementia from classical Alzheimer's disease. Neuroreport 1994;5:747–9.
[36] McKeith IG, Galasko D, Kosaka K, et al. Consensus guidelines for the clinical and pathological diagnosis of dementia with Lewy bodies (DLB): report of the consortium on DLB international workshop. Neurology 1996;47:1113–24.
[37] Shea C, MacKnight C, Rockwood K. Donepezil for treatment of dementia with Lewy bodies: a case series of nine patients. Int Psychogeriatr 1998;10:229–38.
[38] Del Ser T, McKeith I, Anand R, Cicin-Sain A, et al. Dementia with Lewy bodies: findings from an international multicentre study. Int J Geriatr Psychiatry 2000;15:1034–45.
[39] McKeith IG, Perry EK, Perry RH. For the consortium on dementia with Lewy bodies: report of the second dementia with Lewy body international workshop. Neurology 1999;53:902–5.

[40] Keith MS, Stanislav SW, Wesnes KA. Validity of a cognitive computerized assessment system in brain-injured patients. Brain Inj 1998;12:1037–43.

[41] McKeith IG, Del Ser T, Spano P, Emre M, et al. Efficacy of rivastigmine in dementia with Lewy bodies: a randomized, double-blind, placebo-controlled international study. Lancet 2000;356: 2031–6.

[42] Grace J, Daniel S, Stevens T, Shankar KK, et al. Long-term use of rivastigmine in patients with dementia with Lewy bodies: an open-label trial. Int Psychogeriatr 2001;13:199–205.

[43] Rösler M, Cicin-Sain A, Gautheir S, et al. Efficacy and safety of rivastigmine in patients with Alzheimer's disease: international randomised controlled trial. Br Med J 1999;318:633–8.

[44] Skjerve A, Nygaard HA. Improvement in sundowning in dementia with Lewy bodies after treatment with donepezil. Int J Geriatr Psychiatry 2000;15:1147–51.

[45] Kaufer DI, Catt KE, DeKosky ST, et al. Dementia with Lewy bodies: response of delirium like features to donepezil. Neurology 1998;51:1512.

[46] Lanctot K, Herrmann N. Donepezil for behavioural disorders associated with Lewy bodies: a case series. Int J Geriatr Psychiatry 2000;15:338–45.

[47] Tariot PN, Solomon PR, Morris JC, et al. A 5-month, randomized, placebo-controlled trial of galantamine in AD. The Galantamine USA-10 Study Group. Neurology 2000;54(12):2269–76.

[48] Whitehouse PJ, Price DL, Clark AW, Coyle JT, De Long MR. Alzheimer's disease: evidence for selective loss of cholinergic neurons in the nucleus basalis. Ann Neurol 1981;10:122–6.

[49] Giladi N, Shabtai H, Gurevich T, Benbunan B, Anca M, Korczyn AD. Rivastigmine (Exelon) for dementia in patients with Parkinson's disease. Acta Neurol Scand 2003;108(5):368–73.

[50] Reading PJ, Luce AK, McKeith IG. Rivastigmine in the treatment of parkinsonian psychosis and cognitive impairment: preliminary findings from an open trial. Mov Disord 2001;16(6):1171–4.

[51] Aarsland D, Hutchinson M, Larsen JP. Cognitive, psychiatric and motor response to galantamine in Parkinson's disease with dementia. Int J Geriatr Psychiatry 2003;18:937–41.

[52] Aarsland D, Laake K, Larsen JP, Janvin C. Donepezil for cognitive impairment in Parkinson's disease: a randomized controlled study. J Neurol Neurosurg Psychiatry 2002;72:708–12.

ELSEVIER
SAUNDERS

Clin Geriatr Med 20 (2004) 69–82

CLINICS IN
GERIATRIC
MEDICINE

Managing agitation and difficult behavior in dementia

Kevin F. Gray, MD[a,b,*]

[a]*Departments of Psychiatry and Neurology, University of Texas Southwestern Medical Center, 5323 Harry Hines Blvd., Dallas, TX 75235-9070, USA*

[b]*Geriatric Neuropsychiatry Clinic, Veterans Affairs North Texas Health Care System, 4500 South Lancaster Rd., Dallas, TX 75216, USA*

The dementias are associated with disruptions in cognition, function, and behavior. Before the advent of dementia-specific therapies, management of difficult behaviors was the primary "treatment" of demented persons. Problematic behavioral symptoms such as agitation, apathy, depression, anxiety, delusions, irritability, and disinhibition are highly prevalent during the course of dementia [1]. Agitation and difficult behaviors are important factors influencing a family's decision to choose nursing home placement for their demented elder [2]. Agitation occurs in as many as 70% to 90% of demented elderly nursing home patients, perhaps 50% of whom become frankly aggressive [3]. The term "agitation" describes inappropriate verbal, vocal, or motor activity that does not result from need. The agitated behaviors do not serve the interest of the patient and adversely affect others' efforts to help. Some behaviors are inherently inappropriate, whereas others may be inappropriate due to their intensity, frequency, or the context in which they are exhibited [4]. Increasingly, the term "behavioral and psychological symptoms of dementia" is used for clinical purposes to group the myriad agitated and difficult behaviors arising in demented patients [5].

Assessment of agitation and difficult behaviors

It is difficult to directly assess agitation in demented elderly patients, as they are often unable to verbalize their emotions or give reasons for their behavior especially when their dementia is more severe. Agitation assessment methods that

This work was supported by the Department of Veterans Affairs.

* Dallas VA Medical Center (116A), 4500 S. Lancaster Road, Dallas, TX 75216.

E-mail address: Kevin.Gray@med.va.gov

doi:10.1016/j.cger.2003.11.003

rely on direct patient inquiry are generally unreliable in older adults with more than mild to moderate dementia. Observer-based assessment techniques relying on family and staff perspectives are consistently more helpful in accurately characterizing the patient's difficulties and optimizing treatment interventions. This observer-based approach is preferred for more structured research purposes using informant rating scales such as the Cohen-Mansfield Agitation Inventory [6] and the Neuropsychiatric Inventory [7]. For the clinician, appropriate intervention is facilitated by a systematic frame of reference that includes accurate diagnosis (what) and information as to when, where, with whom, how, and how troubling or dangerous agitated or difficult behaviors might be [8].

Clinical interventions must always consider the multifaceted nature of agitation, and when a problem behavior arises, it is helpful to think logically and positively using the mnemonic "IT'S OVER" (see Table 1). First, ***Identify*** the problem behavior; terms like "agitation" may be used nonselectively to describe a very broad range of "unlikable" behaviors. Requesting specific details of the behaviors in question is critical for directing care, and discerning whether the behavior in question is part of a distinct diagnostic syndrome such as delirium or depression may also prove invaluable when selecting interventions. Next the ***Timing*** or frequency of the agitation must be appreciated. Is this a "one-time" occurrence, or is it becoming a regular problem? Is this "sundowning"? Does it occur at a certain time of day, or is it a seemingly random event? Is there an accelerating or "crescendo" quality to the agitation that signals a clear need for intervention? The ***Surroundings*** or environment must be factored into the agitation equation. Is the agitation arising in a structured environment, or does it manifest everywhere? Does overstimulation evoke the problem, or has the patient's environment changed recently? Are there ***Others involved***? Is a familiar caregiver unavailable? Is the "problem" perceived by only a single staff member? Could a new roommate be unsettling for the patient? Is the problem behavior ***Very troubling*** or dangerous? Extreme behaviors call for immediate, powerful responses, whereas more benign behaviors can be observed over time, and interventions can be tailored accordingly. Ideally, some ***Evaluation*** of physical and cognitive status must be used, and sources of pain or discomfort should be identified. Sensory deprivations arising from missing glasses or dysfunctional hearing aids can play a role in problem behaviors. Medications and

Table 1
I-T-S O-V-E-R mnemonic for approaching agitated behaviors in patients with dementia

Mnemonic	Cue	Pertinent question
I	Identify	What is the problem behavior?
T	Timing	When does it happen?
S	Surroundings	Where does it happen?
O	Others involved	Who else is involved?
V	Very troubling	How dangerous is it?
E	Evaluation	What else might be causing it?
R	Recommend	How do I respond?

concurrent medical conditions warrant exploration as potential factors in producing or aggravating agitated behaviors, and in the event of a sudden change in emotional, cognitive, or behavioral status, a physical origin must always be considered. Only after proceeding with assessment in this systematic fashion should therapeutic ***Recommendations*** be made.

Nonpharmacologic principles

American Academy of Neurology practice parameters support the use of first-line nonpharmacologic strategies for agitation, especially when identifiable causes (such as pain) or environmental triggers are responsible [9]. Mastering nonpharmacologic techniques is essential, as clinical experience confirms that various problems such as wandering or purposeless, repetitive activities, or management problems arising from patients with lifelong "difficult personalities" may well prove unresponsive to current pharmacologic interventions. Psychosocial interventions directed toward caregivers, including education, support, and respite care, may improve caregivers' emotional well-being and quality of life. Empowering caregivers with principles of behavioral management may well delay nursing home placement for patients with dementia. At least one controlled study shows that when caregivers are required to join support groups and are supported with ongoing access to individual and family counseling, they are two thirds less likely to place their spouses in nursing homes, particularly during the early to middle stages of dementia when nursing home placement is generally least appropriate [10].

Nonpharmacologic management for dementia caregivers should include the "4-S" elements of Safety, Serenity, Structure, and Sanity (Table 2). ***Safety*** measures similar to "child-proofing" include making sure access to potentially lethal poisons and medications are carefully controlled; firearms, weapons, and "sharps" should be unavailable. Kitchen appliances and power tools are best left unplugged and out of sight. Smoke alarms must be kept in good working order, electric or gas stoves can have "cut-off" switches installed, and water heater temperature should be lowered so that a cognitively impaired bather cannot suffer severe burns, even if only the hot water faucet is operated. Secure locks and fences can limit wandering, and some type of identification, for clothes or per-

Table 2
The "4 S" approach to nonpharmacologic management of agitated behaviors (caregivers can be taught to focus their efforts in these areas to minimize dangerous or disruptive aspects of agitation)

Category	Response
Safety	Control risks—physical, financial, driving
Serenity	Manage affect—avoid overt frustration and anger
Structure	Increase organization—maintain schedules, facilitate good habits
Sanity	Reduce caregiver strain—seek social support, use respite services

son such as an ID bracelet, helps with locating a lost dementia patient. The Alzheimer's Association sponsors Safe Return, a national, government-funded program that assists in the identification and safe, timely return of individuals with dementia who wander off, sometimes far from home, and become lost; caregivers may register their loved ones by phoning (888) 572-8566. Financial safety is enhanced by limiting access to unscrupulous telemarketers; telephones can be silenced, and important messages can be retrieved remotely by caregivers. Similarly, mail can be diverted to a post office box to avoid endless solicitations, while regular monthly bills are converted to automatic or direct pay. Consider limiting television channels to a few favorites and ensuring that shopping channels are blocked. Finally, physicians should ask about and actively discourage driving by demented persons, as a recent evidence-based review found that even mildly demented Alzheimer victims pose a significant traffic safety problem both from crashes and from driving performance measurements [11].

Serenity begins with deliberate and practiced management of affect on the part of the caregiver. As verbal communication becomes increasingly unreliable, the ability to display a pleasant countenance and use a pleasant tone of voice—regardless of the situation—will serve the caregiver well and convey an overall sense of benign circumstance to the demented patient. Speaking directly to the patient in a calm, clear voice accompanied by gentle touching sends unambiguous signals via multiple sensory routes. Communicate affection, provide reassurance, and use simple distractions such as ice cream when levels of tension increase. Regular reminders in the earliest phases of caregiving should stress that logic is increasingly unavailable to the dementia victim, so elaborate explanations and arguments must be avoided. In general, efforts to limit stimuli and avoid sensory overload are important; many demented individuals prefer a certain quiet place with a favorite chair and favorite music. Tapping into available remote memories via reminiscence can be helpful and may allow younger family members more comfortable communications with a demented relative. The office visit is a splendid time for both physician and staff to model appropriate interactions for family caregivers.

Structure and organization of the caregiving routine exploit the capacity of dementia patients to develop and retain new procedural or "habit" memories. Making the environment as regular, predictable, and familiar as possible allows the less impaired implicit memory systems to work in the caregiver's favor [12]. Patience is key and allows new habits—like males urinating while sitting—to be practiced and entrained over time. Scheduled voiding every 2 to 3 hours avoids accidents and allows demented persons and their caregivers to delay the inconvenience of diapering. The physician should emphasize that establishing a routine is a critical, first step for every dementia caregiver; once a consistent routine is in place, the family may make changes gradually, as needed.

Finally, preserving the caregiver's ***Sanity*** allows for optimal patient care, as caregiver "burnout" is a major determinant of nursing home placement [13]. In addition to the added burden of care responsibilities, caregivers often struggle to cope with the loss of intimacy in their relationship with the dementia victim.

Social isolation must be avoided, and the physician may need to foster the enlistment of adult children to relieve burden from an aged spouse, who may feel overwhelmed by the caregiving duties and angered by the criticism implied by family or physician suggestions that changes in care technique might be beneficial. Helping caregivers set limits and reasonable goals, along with regular reminders that "heroic" efforts are neither expected nor desirable, keeps family morale high. Benevolent physician and staff support reinforces caregivers learning to work ***smarter***, not harder, and to ignore benign behaviors; family members must learn to avoid personalizing hurtful or insensitive comments that arise out of the dementia. Imaginative solutions, combined with common sense and loving concern, should always be encouraged.

Other general principles for coping with agitation and difficult behaviors include having fewer expectations for the patient late in the day. Caregivers should be flexible and willing to compromise, knowing when to back off and let the patient relax. "They can't resist if you don't insist" is an important rule when resistance to care becomes an issue. Caregivers ideally will remind and assist rather than take over and foster dependency in the dementia patient. Skill, technique, and timing, rather than the use of brute force, are the essential ingredients for successful caregiving.

Research into optimal nonpharmacologic approaches is ongoing. In 2000, a randomized, placebo-controlled, multicenter trial demonstrated comparable modest reductions in agitated behaviors for both pharmacologic and nonpharmacologic therapies [14], whereas a more recent study found that exercise training combined with teaching caregivers behavioral management techniques improved both physical health and depression in patients with Alzheimer's disease [15]. Nevertheless, implementation of nonpharmacologic principles remains erratic in clinical and institutional practice despite guidelines and recommendations that it be used as a first-line strategy. In a current survey, only half of all outpatient providers implemented caregiver support practices for at least half of their patients [16], and although the use of pharmacologic agents has decreased in nursing homes since the Nursing Home Reform Act of 1987, there is little evidence to suggest that the use of nonpharmacologic interventions has increased [17]. Before initiating pharmacotherapy for difficult behaviors, the clinician must maintain the realistic perspective that neither pharmacologic nor nonpharmacologic interventions totally eliminate behavioral symptoms, but both types of interventions decrease the severity of symptoms [18]. Even when nonpharmacologic techniques are used, pharmacotherapy may be required at some point in ongoing management of agitated behaviors in persons with dementia [19].

Pharmacotherapies

When psychotropic medications are used to manage agitation and difficult behaviors, they should be used judiciously, in the lowest effective doses and for the shortest period of time necessary. Pharmacotherapy must be monitored closely for effectiveness as well as for side effects. Ineffective medications should be stopped, while consideration should be given to periodic trial dose reductions of effective medications to learn whether treatment is still necessary [20]. Diverse classes of psychotropic medication including the cholinesterase inhibitors, antidepressants such as trazodone and the selective serotonin re-uptake inhibitors, and anticonvulsants such as valproic acid have demonstrated efficacy in treating agitation. Antipsychotics are the best studied pharmacologic intervention for agitation and aggression and demonstrate modest but consistent efficacy. Benzodiazepines can be used for short-term agitation treatment as "p.r.n." (as needed) agents when necessary [21].

Cholinesterase inhibitors

Although this is a relatively new class of psychotropic medication approved primarily for cognitive enhancement, studies using cholinesterase inhibitors have demonstrated clear potential to improve or stabilize existing agitation and problem behaviors in dementia [22]. As the three cholinesterase inhibitors most commonly used, donepezil, rivastigmine, and galantamine are the current recommended standard of care for the symptomatic treatment of mild to moderate Alzheimer's disease, early initiation of therapy with one these agents is vital [9]. Except in more urgent or emergent circumstances, evolving clinical practice suggests first observing the impact of cholinesterase inhibitors on behavioral symptoms, as milder disturbances may not require other psychotropic drugs. One recent report recommended that cholinesterase inhibitors be considered for the treatment of problem behaviors before neuroleptic treatment is instituted in Alzheimer patients with low levels of irritability and agitation [23]. Similarly, an earlier study suggested that behavioral responders to cholinesterase inhibitor therapy showed improvement in delusions, agitation, anxiety, disinhibition, and irritability [24]. Consistent findings of benefit for irritability and disinhibition imply that a pretreatment orbitofrontal syndrome may underlie behavioral response to this class of medication in Alzheimer's disease [25], whereas newer studies are demonstrating behavioral benefits in Lewy body and Parkinson's dementias [26,27]. Preliminary observations suggest the potential value of cholinesterase inhibitors in the treatment of psychotic symptoms in dementia patients, with one study suggesting that augmentation of neuroleptics with a cholinesterase inhibitor may be appropriate for patients when neuroleptic monotherapy either does not lead to symptom remission or is associated with intolerable adverse effects [28]. A current meta-analysis found no difference in efficacy among various cholinesterase inhibitors and confirmed their modest beneficial impact on neuropsychiatric and functional outcomes [29].

Antidepressants

Although prevalence estimates of major depression in Alzheimer's disease vary widely from $> 50\%$ to $< 2\%$ [30,31], depressive symptoms are nevertheless common enough to spur development of provisional consensus diagnostic criteria [32]. Although families and other caregivers may interpret the apathy and detachment often accompanying dementia syndromes as "depression," in clinical practice, "low spirits" and dysphoric colorations of mood are commonly reported in dementia patients. Given the benign character of available antidepressant drugs and the curability of depressive symptoms, there is little harm in maintaining a low threshold for initiating a trial of antidepressant medication in dementia patients. Additionally, new research points to altered central serotonergic activity as a contributor to aggressive behaviors in Alzheimer's disease [33].

Selective serotonin re-uptake inhibitors (SSRIs) have well-established efficacy, safety, and tolerability in older patients with depression, including depression secondary to stroke or dementia or other comorbid physical disorders. Citalopram (10 to 40 mg at bedtime) or sertraline (25 to100 mg every morning) are generally preferred agents, as fluoxetine or paroxetine are more likely to be involved in significant drug-drug interactions. In practice, one SSRI may be more efficacious or better tolerated by elderly patients than another, although existing data do not support such claims [34]. The SSRIs show benefit not only for depression and anxiety but also help irritability and mood reactivity; a recent study found citalopram outperformed an antipsychotic for psychosis and behavioral disturbances in nondepressed, demented patients [35].

Trazodone, though little used as primary therapy for depression, remains an important alternative medication for the treatment of behavioral symptoms in dementia patients. In a recent survey of prescribing practices for old age psychiatrists in the United Kingdom, trazodone was the most popular nonneuroleptic medication prescribed for this purpose [36]. A double-blind comparison study found that moderate doses of trazodone (50 to 250 mg/day) and haloperidol (1 to 5 mg/day) were equally effective for treatment of overall agitated behaviors in patients with dementia; although there was no significant difference in improvement between the medication groups, adverse effects were more common with haloperidol. Repetitive, verbally aggressive, and oppositional behaviors responded preferentially to trazodone, whereas symptoms of excessive motor activity and unwarranted accusations responded preferentially to haloperidol [37]. Trazodone is especially useful as an adjunctive medication for sleep facilitation in the elderly. Dosed in the range of 50 to 150 mg at bedtime, it can be given nightly on a long-term basis with good results; elderly patients in well-supervised settings can be given an additional 50 mg during the night as a "p.r.n." for disturbed sleep.

Mirtazapine is a newer agent that shows promise as an effective antidepressant in the elderly. In a comparison trial examining efficacy and tolerability of mirtazapine and paroxetine in elderly patients with major depression, mirtazapine showed an earlier onset of action and also demonstrated a better tolerability profile [38]. These findings, along with a low potential for adverse drug interactions, a tendency to promote appetite and body weight gain, its utility in patients who present with anxiety symptoms and sleep disturbance, and its availability in a rapid-dissolving oral formulation make it an attractive option, especially for infirm or institutionalized elderly. Case reports confirm mirtazapine benefits in depressed Alzheimer patents complicated by weight loss, insomnia, and anxiety [39] as well as remission of new-onset delusional misidentification in an elderly gentleman [40].

Antipsychotics

Psychotic symptoms are common in dementia patients, occurring in 60% of nursing home elders in a recent report [41]. Moreover, psychosis is significantly associated with aggression in dementia [42], and diagnostic criteria have been proposed to further research into the psychosis of dementia syndromes [43]. Antipsychotic medications are modestly effective for the treatment of psychosis and agitation in elderly patients with dementia [44]. In clinical practice, very low doses of the older or conventional neuroleptics may be effective and may limit the development of severe extrapyramidal reactions, although accumulating experience suggests that the newer atypical neuroleptics are also useful for controlling severe agitation in elderly demented patients [45].

Conventional antipsychotics have been used to treat agitation and problematic behaviors in dementia victims for decades. In a landmark meta-analytic review of existing literature, Schneider et al [46] confirmed that conventional neuroleptics are modestly effective (18% better than placebo) in treating dementia-related agitation and further supported the clinical impression that no single neuroleptic was more efficacious than another in this population. Haloperidol remains the most commonly used antipsychotic for control of behavioral and psychologic symptoms of dementia. Dosing varies widely in clinical practice, but a careful double-blind, placebo-controlled trial comparing the efficacy and side effects of two doses of haloperidol and placebo found that standard-dose (2 to 3 mg/day) haloperidol was efficacious and superior to both low-dose (0.50 to 0.75 mg/day) haloperidol and placebo for psychosis and disruptive behaviors in patients with Alzheimer's disease. A starting haloperidol dose of 1 mg/day with gradual, upward dose titration was recommended [47]. One disturbing finding in this study was that extrapyramidal signs tended to be greater with the standard dose, primarily because of a subgroup (20%) who developed moderate to severe signs, thereby rendering overall haloperidol suitability for a dementia population less clear. Emerging studies cast doubt on the traditional role of haloperidol therapy; one such study found that even the presence of delusions in concert with behavioral disturbance did not predict greater behavioral improvement with haloperidol when compared with trazodone [48]. Similarly, a current evidence-based Cochrane Review suggests that haloperidol is useful in the control of aggression but is associated with increased side effects. This review found no evidence to support the routine use of haloperidol for other manifestations of agitated dementia and confirmed that haloperidol should not be used routinely to treat patients with agitated dementia. Instead, treatment of agitated dementia with haloperidol should be individualized, and patients should be monitored for side effects of therapy [49].

Atypical antipsychotics such as risperidone, olanzapine, and quetiapine are emerging as the standard antipsychotics for use in treating behavioral and psychological symptoms of dementia, appearing at least as effective as the conventional agents while having fewer adverse effects. A recent factor analysis of short-term antipsychotic effectiveness in hospitalized dementia patients found that olanzapine and risperidone were as effective as haloperidol for disruptive overactivity, thought/communication disorder, interpersonal aggressiveness, and destructiveness [50]. Similarly, a large, double-blind, placebo-controlled study of institutionalized elderly patients with dementia found that risperidone significantly improved symptoms of psychosis and aggressive behavior and concluded that 1 mg/day of risperidone is an appropriate dose for most elderly patients with dementia [51,52]. Olanzapine in low doses (5 to 10 mg/day) has been shown significantly superior to placebo and well tolerated in treating agitation/aggression and psychosis in elderly US nursing home residents with Alzheimer's disease [53]. Use of orally disintegrating olanzapine is preferred for the acute management of psychobehavioral disturbances in demented patients who resist or have difficulty taking standard oral medications [54]. Clinical trials in agitated younger patients experiencing an acute decompensation of schizophrenia or bipolar disorder show doses up to 40 mg/day may offer superior efficacy in rapidly and effectively controlling the symptoms of agitation [55]. Applying these findings to acute, extreme agitation in our elderly demented patients, we find short-term olanzapine oral loading strategies using 10 to 20 mg/day to be quite helpful. A rapid-acting intramuscular olanzapine formulation has been approved for use in treating agitation associated with dementia but is not yet available for clinical use [56]. Quetiapine is proving to be an important drug for treating psychosis and agitation in Lewy body/Parkinson-spectrum dementias using doses in the 25 to 75 mg/day range [57,58]. Use of quetiapine for behavioral management in Alzheimer's disease is less well established, although one recent case series reports significant diminution of delusions, aggression, and problematic behaviors at doses ranging from 50 to 150 mg/day [59]. Despite a published case series of older patients with psychosis and behavioral disruption [60], use of clozapine is generally reserved for Parkinson's disease patients with psychosis [61]. Finally, although anecdotal reports are promising, published research in demented elders is needed for the recently approved agents, aripiprazole and ziprasidone.

Anticonvulsants

Disenchantment with antipsychotics has fueled a quest for alternative medications to control agitation and problem behaviors associated with dementia. Clinical experience over the past decade has begun to confirm the value of anticonvulsants or "mood stabilizers" for this purpose. Although anecdotal reports abound, systematic studies of valproate/divalproex and carbamazepine are best established. A recent extended trial of divalproex sodium in 56 nursing home patients with agitation and dementia found good tolerability and improvement in measures of agitation in the dose range of 250 to 1500 mg/day (mean: 851 mg/day) [62]. Recent findings suggesting neuroprotective properties for valproate may lead to trials examining whether chronic valproate therapy can attenuate the clinical progression of Alzheimer's disease by delaying or preventing the onset of agitation in patients lacking agitation to begin with, as well as slowing progressive decline in cognition and daily functioning [63]. Although valproate appears to provide a useful option for controlling problem behaviors in individual patients, its routine use may be limited by reports of reversible Parkinsonism and cognitive impairment with chronic therapy [64]. Carbamazepine has been studied in 51 demented nursing home patients and showed significant short-term efficacy for agitation with generally good safety and tolerability. Modal carbamazepine dose at 6 weeks was 300 mg/day, and a mean serum level of 5.3 μg/mL was achieved [65]. Case reports are emerging for gabapentin as a possible treatment of difficult behaviors in dementia [66,67].

Anxiolytics and other agents

Benzodiazepines are commonly prescribed in the elderly, and people with dementia may be at a greater risk of adverse drug reactions such as cognitive impairment. Alzheimer's disease patients are frequently prescribed benzodiazepines, often as a "p.r.n." medication for calming. One recent study found as many as 20% of Alzheimer victims were given benzodiazepines, although progression of dementia was associated with a decreased use of this drug class [68]. Although concerns about mental dulling, falls, and disinhibition of behaviors have limited widespread current use of benzodiazepines, at least one study found alprazolam was equally as effective as low dose haloperidol in managing disruptive behavioral episodes associated with delirium, dementia, and amnesic and other cognitive disorders in nursing home residents [69]. A trial of buspirone for the control of disruptive behaviors in dementia found significant improvement at an optimal starting dosage of 30 mg daily (70). Individual patients may have their best response at dosages ranging from 15 to 60 mg daily [70]. Intramuscular medroxyprogesterone acetate dosed at 150 mg every 2 weeks to every month has proven to be very effective for sexual aggression in elderly men [71]. Because of its safety and efficacy, the drug should be considered as a first-line treatment for sexual acting out in demented men [72].

Summary

Managing agitation and difficult behavior in dementia can be the most challenging aspect of dementia care, as behavioral and psychological symptoms of dementia cause premature institutionalization, increase costs of care, and result in significant loss of quality of life for the patient and the family caregivers. Nonpharmacologic interventions are important first-line steps in dealing with milder symptoms, whereas medication is clearly indicated in conjunction with nonpharmacologic interventions for more severe and problematic behaviors. Various classes of medication, including cholinesterase inhibitors, antidepressants, atypical antipsychotics, anticonvulsants, and anxiolytics represent the reference drugs for treating agitation. Nonetheless, there is no currently available ideal pharmacotherapy.

Acknowledgments

The author gratefully acknowledges the assistance of David S. Geldmacher, MD, in the preparation of this article.

References

[1] Cummings JL, McPherson S. Neuropsychiatric assessment of Alzheimer's disease and related dementias. Aging (Milano) 2001;13(3):240–6.

[2] Steele C, Rovner B, Chase GA, Folstein M. Psychiatric symptoms and nursing home placement of patients with Alzheimer's disease. Am J Psychiatry 1990;147(8):1049–51.

[3] Cohen-Mansfield J. Assessment of agitation. Int Psychogeriatr 1996;8(2):233–45.

[4] Cohen-Mansfield J, Marx MS, Rosenthal AS. A description of agitation in a nursing home. J Gerontol 1989;44(3):M77–84.

[5] Finkel SI. Behavioral and psychological symptoms of dementia: a current focus for clinicians, researchers, and caregivers. J Clin Psychiatry 2001;62(Suppl 21):3–6.

[6] Koss E, Weiner M, Ernesto C, Cohen-Mansfield J, Ferris SH, Grundman M, et al. Assessing patterns of agitation in Alzheimer's disease patients with the Cohen-Mansfield Agitation Inventory. The Alzheimer's Disease Cooperative Study. Alzheimer Dis Assoc Disord 1997; 11(Suppl 2): S45–50.

[7] Cummings JL, Mega M, Gray KF, Rosenberg-Thompson S, Carusi DA, Gornbein J. The neuropsychiatric inventory: comprehensive assessment of psychopathology in dementia. Neurology 1994;44(12):2308–14.

[8] Weiner MF, Gray KF. Balancing psychosocial and psychopharmacologic measures in Alzheimer's disease. Am J Alzheimers Care Related Disord Res 1994;9(4):6–12.

[9] Doody RS, Stevens JC, Beck C, Dubinsky RM, Kaye JA, Gwyther L, et al. Practice parameter: management of dementia (an evidence-based review). Report of the Quality Standards Subcommittee of the American Academy of Neurology. Neurology 2001;56(9):1154–66.

[10] Mittelman MS, Ferris SH, Shulman E, Steinberg G, Levin B. A family intervention to delay nursing home placement of patients with Alzheimer disease. A randomized controlled trial [see comments]. JAMA 1996;276(21):1725–31.

[11] Dubinsky RM, Stein AC, Lyons K. Practice parameter: risk of driving and Alzheimer's disease (an evidence-based review): report of the Quality Standards Subcommittee of the American Academy of Neurology. Neurology 2000;54(12):2205–11.

[12] De Vreese LP, Neri M, Fioravanti M, Belloi L, Zanetti O. Memory rehabilitation in Alzheimer's disease: a review of progress. Int J Geriatr Psychiatry 2001;16(8):794–809.

[13] Hebert R, Dubois MF, Wolfson C, Chambers L, Cohen C. Factors associated with long-term institutionalization of older people with dementia: data from the Canadian Study of Health and Aging. J Gerontol A Biol Sci Med Sci 2001;56(11):M693–9.

[14] Teri L, Logsdon RG, Peskind E, Raskind M, Weiner MF, Tractenberg RE, et al. Treatment of agitation in AD: a randomized, placebo-controlled clinical trial. Neurology 2000;55(9):1271–8.

[15] Teri L, Gibbons LE, McCurry SM, Logsdon RG, Buchner DM, Barlow WE, et al. Exercise plus behavioral management in patients with Alzheimer disease: a randomized controlled trial. JAMA 2003;290(15):2015–22.

[16] Rosen CS, Chow HC, Greenbaum MA, Finney JF, Moos RH, Sheikh JI, et al. How well are clinicians following dementia practice guidelines? Alzheimer Dis Assoc Disord 2002;16(1): 15–23.

[17] Cody M, Beck C, Svarstad BL. Challenges to the use of nonpharmacologic interventions in nursing homes. Psychiatr Serv 2002;53(11):1402–6.

[18] Snowden M, Sato K, Roy-Byrne P. Assessment and treatment of nursing home residents with depression or behavioral symptoms associated with dementia: a review of the literature. J Am Geriatr Soc 2003;51(9):1305–17.

[19] Weiner MF, Tractenberg RE, Sano M, Logsdon R, Teri L, Galasko D, et al. No long-term effect of behavioral treatment on psychotropic drug use for agitation in Alzheimer's disease patients. J Geriatr Psychiatry Neurol 2002;15(2):95–8.

[20] Tariot P, Gaile SE, Castelli NA, Porsteinsson AP. Treatment of agitation in dementia. New Dir Ment Health Serv 1997;76:109–23.

[21] Herrmann N. Recommendations for the management of behavioral and psychological symptoms of dementia. Can J Neurol Sci 2001;28(Suppl 1):S96–107.

[22] Grossberg GT. The ABC of Alzheimer's disease: behavioral symptoms and their treatment. Int Psychogeriatr 2002;14(Suppl 1):27–49.

[23] Paleacu D, Mazeh D, Mirecki I, Even M, Barak Y. Donepezil for the treatment of behavioral symptoms in patients with Alzheimer's disease. Clin Neuropharmacol 2002;25(6):313–7.

[24] Mega MS, Masterman DM, O'Connor SM, Barclay TR, Cummings JL. The spectrum of behavioral responses to cholinesterase inhibitor therapy in Alzheimer disease. Arch Neurol 1999; 56(11):1388–93.

[25] Mega MS, Dinov ID, Lee L, O'Connor SM, Masterman DM, Wilen B, et al. Orbital and dorsolateral frontal perfusion defect associated with behavioral response to cholinesterase inhibitor therapy in Alzheimer's disease. J Neuropsychiatry Clin Neurosci 2000;12(2):209–18.

[26] Lanctot KL, Herrmann N. Donepezil for behavioural disorders associated with Lewy bodies: a case series. Int J Geriatr Psychiatry 2000;15(4):338–45.

[27] Aarsland D, Hutchinson M, Larsen JP. Cognitive, psychiatric and motor response to galantamine in Parkinson's disease with dementia. Int J Geriatr Psychiatry 2003;18(10):937–41.

[28] Bergman J, Brettholz I, Shneidman M, Lerner V. Donepezil as add-on treatment of psychotic symptoms in patients with dementia of the Alzheimer's type. Clin Neuropharmacol 2003;26(2): 88–92.

[29] Trinh NH, Hoblyn J, Mohanty S, Yaffe K. Efficacy of cholinesterase inhibitors in the treatment of neuropsychiatric symptoms and functional impairment in Alzheimer disease: a meta-analysis. JAMA 2003;289(2):210–6.

[30] Zubenko GS, Zubenko WN, McPherson S, Spoor E, Marin DB, Farlow MR, et al. A collaborative study of the emergence and clinical features of the major depressive syndrome of Alzheimer's disease. Am J Psychiatry 2003;160(5):857–66.

[31] Weiner MF, Edland SD, Luszczynska H. Prevalence and incidence of major depression in Alzheimer's disease. Am J Psychiatry 1994;151(7):1006–9.

[32] Olin JT, Schneider LS, Katz IR, Meyers BS, Alexopoulos GS, Breitner JC, et al. Provisional diagnostic criteria for depression of Alzheimer disease. Am J Geriatr Psychiatry 2002; 10(2):125–8.

[33] Lanctot KL, Herrmann N, Van Reekum R, Eryavec G, Naranjo CA. Gender, aggression and serotonergic function are associated with response to sertraline for behavioral disturbances in Alzheimer's disease. Int J Geriatr Psychiatry 2002;17(6):531–41.

[34] Solai LK, Mulsant BH, Pollock BG. Selective serotonin reuptake inhibitors for late-life depression: a comparative review. Drugs Aging 2001;18(5):355–68.

[35] Pollock BG, Mulsant BH, Rosen J, Sweet RA, Mazumdar S, Bharucha A, et al. Comparison of citalopram, perphenazine, and placebo for the acute treatment of psychosis and behavioral disturbances in hospitalized, demented patients. Am J Psychiatry 2002;159(3):460–5.

[36] Condren RM, Cooney C. Use of drugs by old age psychiatrists in the treatment of psychotic and behavioural symptoms in patients with dementia. Aging Ment Health 2001;5(3):235–41.

[37] Sultzer DL, Gray KF, Gunay I, Berisford MA, Mahler ME. A double-blind comparison of trazodone and haloperidol for treatment of agitation in patients with dementia. Am J Geriatr Psychiatry 1997;5(1):60–9.
[38] Schatzberg AF, Kremer C, Rodrigues HE, Murphy Jr JG. The mirtazapine vs paroxetine study group. Double-blind, randomized comparison of mirtazapine and paroxetine in elderly depressed patients. Am J Geriatr Psychiatry 2002;10(5):541–50.
[39] Raji MA, Brady SR. Mirtazapine for treatment of depression and comorbidities in Alzheimer disease. Ann Pharmacother 2001;35(9):1024–7.
[40] Khouzam HR. Capgras syndrome responding to the antidepressant mirtazapine. Compr Ther 2002;28(3):238–40.
[41] Brodaty H, Draper B, Saab D, Low LF, Richards V, Paton H, et al. Psychosis, depression and behavioural disturbances in Sydney nursing home residents: prevalence and predictors. Int J Geriatr Psychiatry 2001;16(5):504–12.
[42] Rapoport MJ, Van Reekum R, Freedman M, Streiner D, Simard M, Clarke D, et al. Relationship of psychosis to aggression, apathy and function in dementia. Int J Geriatr Psychiatry 2001; 16(2):123–30.
[43] Jeste DV, Finkel SI. Psychosis of Alzheimer's disease and related dementias. Diagnostic criteria for a distinct syndrome. Am J Geriatr Psychiatry 2000;8(1):29–34.
[44] Kindermann SS, Dolder CR, Bailey A, Katz IR, Jeste DV. Pharmacological treatment of psychosis and agitation in elderly patients with dementia: four decades of experience. Drugs Aging 2002;19(4):257–76.
[45] Salzman C. Treatment of the agitation of late-life psychosis and Alzheimer's disease. Eur Psychiatry 2001;16(Suppl 1):25–8.
[46] Schneider LS, Pollock VE, Lyness SA. A metaanalysis of controlled trials of neuroleptic treatment in dementia. J Am Geriatr Soc 1990;38:553–63.
[47] Devanand DP, Marder K, Michaels KS, Sackeim HA, Bell K, Sullivan MA, et al. A randomized, placebo-controlled dose-comparison trial of haloperidol for psychosis and disruptive behaviors in Alzheimer's disease. Am J Psychiatry 1998;155(11):1512–20.
[48] Sultzer DL, Gray KF, Gunay I, Wheatley MV, Mahler ME. Does behavioral improvement with haloperidol or trazodone treatment depend on psychosis or mood symptoms in patients with dementia? J Am Geriatr Soc 2001;49(10):1294–300.
[49] Lonergan E, Luxenberg J, Colford J. Haloperidol for agitation in dementia (Cochrane Review). Cochrane Database Syst Rev 2002;(2):CD002852.
[50] Adams BE, Tunis SL, Edell WS. Assessing antipsychotic effectiveness in dementia with the factor structure of the psychogeriatric dependency rating scale (PGDRS). J Am Med Dir Assoc 2003;4(2):61–6.
[51] Katz IR, Jeste DV, Mintzer JE, Clyde C, Napolitano J, Brecher M. Comparison of risperidone and placebo for psychosis and behavioral disturbances associated with dementia: a randomized, double-blind trial. Risperidone Study Group. J Clin Psychiatry 1999;60(2):107–15.
[52] Schneider LS, Katz IR, Park S, Napolitano J, Martinez RA, Azen SP. Psychosis of Alzheimer disease: validity of the construct and response to risperidone. Am J Geriatr Psychiatry 2003; 11(4):414–25.
[53] Street JS, Clark WS, Gannon KS, Cummings JL, Bymaster FP, Tamura RN, et al. Olanzapine treatment of psychotic and behavioral symptoms in patients with Alzheimer disease in nursing care facilities: a double-blind, randomized, placebo-controlled trial. The HGEU Study Group. Arch Gen Psychiatry 2000;57(10):968–76.
[54] Reeves RR, Torres RA. Orally disintegrating olanzapine for the treatment of psychotic and behavioral disturbances associated with dementia. South Med J 2003;96(7):699–701.
[55] Baker RW, Kinon BJ, Maguire GA, Liu H, Hill AL. Effectiveness of rapid initial dose escalation of up to forty milligrams per day of oral olanzapine in acute agitation. J Clin Psychopharmacol 2003;23(4):342–8.
[56] Meehan KM, Wang H, David SR, Nisivoccia JR, Jones B, Beasley CM, et al. Comparison of rapidly acting intramuscular olanzapine, lorazepam, and placebo. A double-blind, random-

ized study in acutely agitated patients with dementia. Neuropsychopharmacology 2002;26(4): 494–504.

[57] Fernandez HH, Trieschmann ME, Burke MA, Jacques C, Friedman JH. Long-term outcome of quetiapine use for psychosis among parkinsonian patients. Mov Disord 2003;18(5):510–4.

[58] Takahashi H, Yoshida K, Sugita T, Higuchi H, Shimizu T. Quetiapine treatment of psychotic symptoms and aggressive behavior in patients with dementia with Lewy bodies: a case series. Prog Neuropsychopharmacol Biol Psychiatry 2003;27(3):549–53.

[59] Scharre DW, Chang SI. Cognitive and behavioral effects of quetiapine in Alzheimer disease patients. Alzheimer Dis Assoc Disord 2002;16(2):128–30.

[60] Salzman C, Vaccaro B, Lieff J, Weiner A. Clozapine in older patients with psychosis and behavioral disruption. Am J Geriatr Psychiatry 1995;3(1):26–33.

[61] Klein C, Gordon J, Pollak L, Rabey JM. Clozapine in Parkinson's disease psychosis: 5-year follow-up review. Clin Neuropharmacol 2003;26(1):8–11.

[62] Porsteinsson AP, Tariot PN, Jakimovich LJ, Kowalski N, Holt C, Erb R, et al. Valproate therapy for agitation in dementia: open-label extension of a double-blind trial. Am J Geriatr Psychiatry 2003;11(4):434–40.

[63] Tariot PN, Loy R, Ryan JM, Porsteinsson A, Ismail S. Mood stabilizers in Alzheimer's disease: symptomatic and neuroprotective rationales. Adv Drug Deliv Rev 2002;54(12):1567–77.

[64] Armon C, Shin C, Miller P, Carwile S, Brown E, Edinger JD, et al. Reversible parkinsonism and cognitive impairment with chronic valproate use. Neurology 1996;47(3):626–35.

[65] Tariot PN, Erb R, Podgorski CA, Cox C, Patel S, Jakimovich L, et al. Efficacy and tolerability of carbamazepine for agitation and aggression in dementia. Am J Psychiatry 1998;155(1): 54–61.

[66] Miller LJ. Gabapentin for treatment of behavioral and psychological symptoms of dementia. Ann Pharmacother 2001;35(4):427–31.

[67] Hawkins JW, Tinklenberg JR, Sheikh JI, Peyser CE, Yesavage JA. A retrospective chart review of gabapentin for the treatment of aggressive and agitated behavior in patients with dementias. Am J Geriatr Psychiatry 2000;8(3):221–5.

[68] Lagnaoui R, Moore N, Moride Y, Miremont-Salame G, Begaud B. Benzodiazepine utilization patterns in Alzheimer's disease patients. Pharmacoepidemiol Drug Saf 2003;12(6):511–5.

[69] Christensen DB, Benfield WR. Alprazolam as an alternative to low-dose haloperidol in older, cognitively impaired nursing facility patients. J Am Geriatr Soc 1998;46(5):620–5.

[70] Cooper JP. Buspirone for anxiety and agitation in dementia. J Psychiat Neurosci 2003;28(6):469.

[71] Weiner MF, Denke M, Williams K, Guzman R. Intramuscular medroxyprogesterone acetate for sexual aggression in elderly men [letter]. Lancet 1992;339(May 2):1121–2.

[72] Cooper AJ. Medroxyprogesterone acetate (MPA) treatment of sexual acting out in men suffering from dementia. J Clin Psychiatry 1987;48(9):368–70.

ELSEVIER
SAUNDERS

Clin Geriatr Med 20 (2004) 83–92

CLINICS IN
GERIATRIC
MEDICINE

Managing dementia in long-term care settings

Suzanne Holroyd, MD

Department of Psychiatric Medicine, University of Virginia HSC, Box 800623, Charlottesville, VA 22908, USA

The majority of patients in long-term care settings (nursing homes) have a diagnosis of dementia. Dementia is associated with a high prevalence of behavioral and psychiatric disorders. In fact, behavioral and psychiatric symptoms of dementia are the major reason patients are placed in long-term care settings [1]. Symptoms such as psychosis, depression, and agitation including aggressiveness, can be overwhelming to patients, families, and staff alike. These difficult symptoms may lead to overmedication with limited benefit and potential side effects. Improved management of patients suffering from dementia can lead to marked improvements for patients, families, and staff, leading to greater optimism and quality of life. In fact, treating this population can be extremely rewarding. This article reviews the management of dementia patients in the long-term care setting, with a focus on correctly diagnosing the reasons for behavioral problems and appropriate treatment strategies

Magnitude of the problem

Until the early 1990s, the prevalence of dementia and psychiatric disorders in the nursing home setting was unknown. Rovner et al [2] first studied the prevalence of dementia and psychiatric disorders in nursing homes. This research revealed that 80.2% of nursing home admissions had a psychiatric disorder, the most common diagnosis (67.4%) being dementia. Of the demented patients, fully 40% had noncognitive psychiatric symptoms as part of their dementia such as psychosis or depression.

Other researchers have similarly found high rates of dementia in nursing homes [3,4], and the rates of behavioral and psychiatric comorbidity also to be high. For example, behavioral problems have been found to occur in 64% to 90% of all

This work supported in part by NIH-R01 NS045008-01A1.

E-mail address: sh4s@virginia.edu

0749-0690/04/$ – see front matter
doi:10.1016/j.cger.2003.10.005

nursing home residents [3,5]. Surprisingly, behavioral problems of dementia do not correlate with the degree of cognitive decline [6]. In fact, although functional changes are closely associated to cognitive decline in dementing illness, behavioral and psychiatric symptoms are not, evidence that the behavioral problems are a distinct syndrome of dementia [7]. Nursing homes now function as "long-term psychiatric hospitals for the elderly" [8]. Nonetheless, the care of such patients typically is managed by internists or family practitioners. As well, care occurs in facilities where the staffing is usually inadequate to deal with such problems; for example, facilities may have only one registered nurse per 49 residents [9].

The types of behavioral and psychiatric disturbances vary greatly from patient to patient and may vary within the same patient. Common symptoms include psychosis, depression, anxiety, insomnia, and agitation including aggressiveness, nondirectable behaviors, and repetitive behaviors. In general, behavioral disturbances peak in the middle stages of dementia, although some specific behaviors increase with worsening dementia [10]. For example, wandering, repeating questions, and psychosis peak in middle dementia, whereas general noisiness and temper outbursts/aggression peak in severe stages of dementia [10]. Psychotic symptoms such as delusions and hallucinations are prevalent in dementia, and they have been best studied in Alzheimer's disease (AD). Although psychosis occurs throughout the course of AD, it is most common at a moderate level of dementia [11].

Delusions are present in 38% to 73% of patients with AD, with paranoid delusions the most common [12,13]. A common paranoid delusion is that of "stealing" things. Studies have shown that the cognition of patients with stealing delusions is not different than those without stealing delusions, supporting that the delusions are not simply due to decreased cognition and the patient's attempt to explain misplaced items [13]. Other common delusions are the "residence is not home" delusion (15% of patients), "infidelity of caregiver" delusion (6%), and "spouse is imposter" delusion in 9% [11,14].

Hallucinations in AD are most commonly visual, occurring in 12% to 53% of AD patients, followed by auditory hallucinations in 6% to 34% [12–15]. Many patients suffer from both delusions and hallucinations. A longitudinal study of psychotic patients with AD revealed that in fact most had both delusions and hallucinations (41%), whereas 23.5% had only delusions and 35.5% had only hallucinations [12].

Importantly, psychosis has been found to be significantly associated with physical aggression in AD patients [16,17]. However, only 23.1% of delusional patients on admission to a nursing home had psychiatric treatment before admission, emphasizing the need to treat psychotic symptoms as a possible cause of aggression and prevention of institutionalization in patients with dementia [18].

Depression is extremely common but underdiagnosed in the demented patient, whether in a long-term care facility or elsewhere. In nursing homes, only 6% to 10% of patients who have depression are actually treated with antidepressants [19,20]. Unfortunately, more patients with depression are treated inappropriately with drugs such as neuroleptics or benzodiazepines [19]. The prevalence of depression in nursing homes is higher than that in community settings, with prevalence in nursing homes of major depression at 20% and clinically significant depressive symptoms another 25% to 40% [21–23].

The prevalence of depression among nursing home residents with dementia is more difficult to estimate, as diagnosis of depression in dementia patients is difficult to establish for several reasons. First, the presence of dementia may change a patient's ability to recognize or communicate typical symptoms of depression, with such abstract concepts of mood, hopelessness, worthlessness, and anhedonia requiring more sophisticated cognitive and language skills. Depression among the demented may thus not meet research criteria for depression. Therefore, the literature of depression in dementia varies, but most studies support that dementia patients have high rates of depression [24–28].

Depression in the elderly may be especially difficult to diagnose. Because symptoms are often not classic for depression, patients are typically misdiagnosed and either not treated at all or treated inappropriately. Depression may simply present as social withdrawal, with patients refusing activities and staying in bed, which they may do politely with seemingly good reason. Patients may refuse irritably (thus ensuring that others may try less in the future to get them to activities again). Severe anxiety [29], agitation, and even extreme aggressive behaviors [30,31] may be the presenting symptom. If one imagines the depressed patient feeling terrible and being unable to articulate that, it becomes easier to understand how aggression and irritability are common symptoms of depression in nursing home settings. Unfortunately, because such symptoms are so prominent for caregivers, depressive symptoms are overlooked and the patient may be treated inappropriately with neuroleptics or sedatives. Similarly, somatic symptoms such as chronic pain [32,33] or over focus on bowels and other physical functioning may be symptoms of depression [34,35]. Tearfulness and decreased appetite with weight loss are often indicative of depression among the demented [36,37].

Evaluation of dementia patients with behavioral or psychiatric disorders

If at all possible, evaluation and treatment of a patient in a nursing home should occur in the nursing home setting. That way, the treating physician can observe the patient in their natural surrounding, giving them a better idea of the problems and solutions. Bringing a dementia patient into an office setting may dramatically alter the presentation of the patient, giving the physician an inaccurate sense of the patient's difficulty. Treating the patient in the nursing home setting also allows for collection of information about the patient from a variety of individuals who work with the patient.

When working with patients in nursing homes, many different and contradictory versions of the patient's behavior can be reported. In the ideal setting, the physician will work in a particular home over a period of time and gain a sense of who the best informants are regarding patients' behaviors. Informants may be the nurses, involved administrators, nursing assistants, physical or occupational therapists, family, or even other patients who may provide useful information.

One of the first steps is defining and establishing that there indeed is a problem. Insist on learning specifics of the problem behavior or concern. The term "agitation" can include a range of behaviors from tapping the table repeatedly or occasionally resisting care to combative or aggressive behaviors such as kicking or choking. Ask for specifics of the behavior: "When you say the patient does not sleep, do you mean he actually does not sleep at all or just doesn't sleep all night? How many hours does he sleep? What is he doing at night when he is awake? When you say the patient is aggressive, what exactly does the patient do?" Make sure to find out when the behaviors started and time of day or activity when they occur and their frequency. Always ask about sleep, appetite, and whether the patient ever cries or seems depressed.

When a patient in a long-term care setting is referred for behavioral problems, the wide range of possibilities for the cause of the problem and the options for treatment can be difficult for the treating physician. In our experience of evaluating patients in the nursing home setting, having a structured order of thinking about the symptoms has helped in defining the diagnostic and treatment possibilities.

The first level is considering the environment in contributing to the behavioral symptom. The second level is considering the medical causes contributing to the behavioral symptom. The third level is considering psychiatric causes contributing to the behavioral symptom. The fourth level is considering the behavioral symptoms as directly due to the dementia itself.

Environmental causes

Environmental causes can sometimes be the most difficult to ascertain but are of utmost importance. Asking about any recent changes in the resident's life (new roommate, family members out of town who usually visit, change of caregiver, loss of a prize possession) is necessary. Sometimes a physician who regularly frequents a particular nursing home will become aware that certain staff always have trouble with residents but other staff working with the same patient do not. A difference in approach to the patient makes all the difference in a patient's willingness to take medication or cooperate with dressing and showering. Other staff may even explain why the other staff member is noting certain behaviors but no one else is. Such information can be extremely useful, and the solutions may simply be change of assignments in consultation with supervising staff. Environmental causes often have environmental solutions, avoiding the mistake of inappropriate prescribing.

Example 1

A referral was made for a 78-year-old woman who had started throwing food at staff and tearing up her towels. She also almost constantly moaned. The symptoms were presented initially by several staff in isolation to any other changes. As the consultant was reviewing the chart, a nursing assistant advised that she thought the patient had gotten worse since getting a new roommate who was quite rude and made constant derogatory statements to the patient. Further questioning revealed the new roommate had made several moves due to difficulty with roommates and indeed had been constantly verbally insulting the patient. The solution was to get a psychiatric referral for the rude roommate and to move her to a private room where she could not to bother others. The throwing food, tearing towels, and moaning behaviors stopped the day after the roommate left.

Example 2

An 83-year-old woman was referred for making a homicidal threat toward a roommate. Further questioning of staff revealed the patient had a new roommate who was extremely demanding and asking for constant help. The patient, who was by history a caring individual, was constantly trying to help the roommate, but she herself had dementia and limited coping abilities to set limits on the roommate's constant requests for help. Finally, one night, the patient could not sleep due to the roommate's constant requests and in frustration threatened to kill the roommate as her only coping mechanism to put an end to the requests. As the pieces of the recent history came into focus, the obvious solution was to move the patient to another room, where she has done beautifully for several years without further aggression or homicidal threats.

Example 3

A 92-year-old woman was referred for constant cursing, irritability, and refusing medication. The referring nurse gave details of the patient's behaviors. Further questioning of other staff working with the patient however revealed the patient has always been irritable but interacting with her in a humorous way resulted in patient cooperation, whereas interacting in a commanding way elicited the undesirable behaviors. Discussing this information with the director of nursing allowed the referring nurse to learn about other ways to interact with the patient.

Medical causes

The next level considers medical causes for behavioral symptoms. Any medication or medical condition has the potential to cause changes in behavior and cognition in patients with dementia. Concomitant medical illness such as urinary tract infections, pneumonia, congestive heart failure, or chronic obstructive pulmonary disease (COPD) exacerbations can be associated with behavioral problems such as poor sleep or appetite, crying, aggressive behaviors, or psychosis. Medications such as narcotics or benzodiazepines, antiparkinson drugs, certain antibiotics, and steroids often cause behavioral problems in demented patients. The patient should be examined carefully for any new medical symptoms that require further investigation or any recent change in medication. Acute pain should also be considered as a medical cause for behavioral problems. A common problem that should always be considered is the urinary tract infection (UTI), and a urinalysis (UA) is warranted for any change in behavior. If a UTI is found, it should be treated even in absence of fever or clear urinary symptoms. Some primary care doctors will not treat a UTI unless there is a fever, making the UTI "symptomatic." In dementia patients, the behavioral change is the symptom of the UTI. Recent stroke or hip fracture patients commonly come to skilled nursing home beds with behavioral problems often due to UTI (had a Foley catheter while in hospital) or narcotics (which can usually be discontinued and nonnarcotic pain relievers substituted).

Example 4

An 80-year-old woman was referred for visual hallucinations of children in her room, poor sleep, and frequent screaming for 2 weeks. Inspection of the patient's legs revealed marked swelling and tenderness of the left leg only. Referral to the emergency room revealed a painful deep venous thrombosis (DVT). When the patient returned after hospitalization for the DVT, there were no behavioral problems.

Example 5

A 75-year-old woman was referred for delusions that her grandson was being hanged by staff and babies were being burned alive. UA revealed a severe UTI, and symptoms resolved several days after treatment for the UTI was started.

Psychiatric causes

The next level considers psychiatric comorbidity as contributing to the behavioral problem. A patient with depression can present with extreme agitation or aggression. Carefully assessing each patient by interview of the patient, multiple staff, and family may elicit depressive symptoms that had gone unnoticed. Treatment with antidepressants instead of other agents may solve a variety of seemingly unrelated behavioral problems. Other psychiatric diagnoses to consider include history of schizophrenia, bipolar disorder, history of recurrent depression, delusional disorder, or anxiety disorders such as obsessive compulsive disorder (OCD) or panic disorder. Treatment specific to these disorders will usually treat the behavior attributed to dementia by staff.

Example 6

An 81-year-old man was referred for extreme irritability, trying to choke staff during caregiving, sudden screaming and cursing, and throwing objects. He paced the hallways and could not be redirected. Examination of the patient revealed he felt sad and wished he were dead. He did not answer other questions regarding depression. Treatment with an antidepressant ended the behaviors within 2 weeks, and he became a favorite patient of staff.

Example 7

A 69-year-old woman with end-stage dementia caused no behavioral problems but had stopped eating and was losing significant weight. The patient was mute on examination, kept her eyes closed, and did not follow any 1 step commands. Assuming possible depression, treatment with antidepressants not only restored her appetite, but she began to smile, hold chatty conversations to the delight of family and staff, and participate in activities long thought too advanced for her.

Example 8

A 74-year-old man was referred for refusal to bathe and eat. History obtained by family revealed a probably history of OCD, never treated, but manifested by overconcern of germs, excessive washing, and specific ways of doing tasks. Although the patient had moderate dementia, allowing him some control in how to do tasks helped partially, but medication aimed at OCD resolved most of the behavior problems.

Behavioral symptoms caused by dementia

The final level considers behaviors to be due to the dementia process itself, which should only be assumed if environmental, medical, and psychiatric levels are evaluated and found to be negative. Treatment for behavioral problems in demented patients should never be an automatic prescription of medication, unless all previous levels have been assessed. If the behaviors are indeed felt to be due to dementia itself, then a treatment guideline can be given. First, decide if the patient is psychotic or not. If the patient is psychotic (hallucinations or delusions), he or she will need antipsychotic treatment, usually with a newer atypical antipsychotic such as olanzapine or quetiapine fumarate. Risperidone, previously used in dementia patients for behavioral disturbances [38,39], has had recent US Food & Drug Administration warnings about possible association with increased risk of stroke [40] and should be avoided, if for no other reason than legal, until more information is gathered.

If patients are not psychotic, the symptom may suggest the treatment. Dementia patients must sleep to have behaviorally normal days. Thus, medication for sleep such as trazadone may be used for a patient having trouble sleeping. Other sleeping aids may be zolpidem or mirtazapine. Avoid benzodiazepines, which are addictive, sedating, and may add to confusion, fall risk, and disinhibited behavior. If all else fails, antipsychotic medications such as olanzapine or quetiapine fumarate may be used to induce sleep but need to be observed carefully for side effects.

If a patient is nonpsychotic and is sleeping well, then a medication such as buspirone can be used to decrease general irritability, agitation, and aggressive/combative behaviors. Mood stabilizers such as divalproex sodium or lithium can be used in mood labile patients and in those for whom the previous trials (buspirone, antipsychotics) have not been successful. Caution must be used, and blood levels and associated blood work must be monitored for side effects (liver function tests, platelet levels for divalproex and thyroid function tests, renal tests for lithium) every 2 to 4 months. Levels should be on the low side for lithium in most cases (0.2 to 0.4) and low to low-therapeutic for divalproex. Free divalproex levels should be done as regular levels may not reveal toxicity in older patients. Because of these monitoring concerns and the potential for side effects, mood stabilizers should only be used if other strategies have failed.

A specialist in geriatric psychiatry may be useful in these evaluations, and it is not uncommon that combinations of the above medications may be needed to address different symptoms (pyschosis, insomnia, depression). The prescribing physician needs to carefully monitor for side effects of the medications especially sedation and change in gait.

For the patient who refuses medication and also refuses medication crushed or hidden in food, medications available in suspension or syrup form may be used. For example, olanzapine is available in an instantly dissolvable form. Sertraline is an antidepressant available in suspension form. Both lithium and divalproex are also available as liquid. In most cases, some strategy can be found to accommodate these patients.

Summary

Treating patients with dementia in the nursing home setting is challenging but extremely rewarding. Satisfaction can be achieved by accurately determining the causes of behavioral problems and formulating treatment plans that work. It is always a good feeling to return to a facility where family and staff are pleased by positive changes in the patient. However, some patients remain difficult to treat despite thorough evaluations and optimal treatment strategies. More research is needed to further define behavioral symptoms of dementia and develop new and effective treatments.

References

[1] Balestreri L, Grossberg A, Grossberg GT. Behavioral and psychological symptoms of dementia as a risk factor for nursing home placement. Int Psychogeriatr 2000;12(Suppl 1):59–62.

[2] Rovner BW, German PS, Broadhead J. The prevalence and management of dementia and other psychiatric disorders in nursing homes. Int Psychogeriatr 1990;2:13–24.

[3] Tariot PN, Podgorski CA, Blazina L, Leibovici A. Mental disorders in the nursing home: another perspective. Am J Psychiatry 1993;150:1063.

[4] Chandler JD, Chandler JE. The prevalence of neuropsychiatric disorders in a nursing home population. J Geriatr Psychiatry Neurol 1998;1:71.

[5] Zimmer JG, Watason NM, Levenson SA. Nursing home medical directors: ideals and realities. J Am Geriatr Soc 1993;41:127–30.

[6] McShane R. What are the syndromes of behavioral and psychological symptoms of dementia? Int Geriatr 2000;12(Suppl 1):147–53.

[7] Finkel SI, Burns A. Introduction–Behavioral and psychological symptoms of dementia (BPSD): a clinical and research update. Int Psychogeriatr 2000;12(Suppl 1):9–12.

[8] Kim E, Rovner BW. The nursing home as a psychiatric hospital. In: Reichman WE, Katz PR, editors. Psychiatric care in the nursing home. New York: Oxford University Press; 1996. p. 3–9.

[9] Mezey M, Knapp M. Nursing staffing in nursing facilities: implications for achieving quality of

care. In: Katz PR, Kane RL, Mezey N, editors. Advances in long term care II. New York: Springer; 1993.
[10] O'Connor DW. Epidemiology of behavioral and psychological symptoms of dementia. Int Psychogeriatr 2000;12(Suppl 1):41–6.
[11] Drevets WC, Rubin EH. Psychotic symptoms and the longitudinal course of senile dementia of the Alzheimer type. Biol Psychiatry 1989;25:39–48.
[12] Lopez OL, Becker JT, Brenner RP. Alzheimer's disease with delusions and hallucinations: neuropsychological and electroencephalographic correlates. Neurology 1991;44:906–12.
[13] Patterson MB, Schnell AH, Martin RJ. Assessment of behavioral and affective symptoms I Alzheimer's disease. J Geriatr Psychiatry Neurol 1990;3:21–30.
[14] Reisberg B, Borenstein J, Salob SP. Behavioral symptoms in Alzheimer's disease: phenomenology and treatment. J Clin Psychiatry 1987;48(Suppl):9–15.
[15] Burns A, Jacoby R, Levy R. Psychiatric phenomena in Alzheimer's disease: II. Disorders of perception. Br J Psychiatry 1990;157:76–81.
[16] Deutsch LH, Bylsma FW, Rovner BW. Psychosis and physical aggression in probable Alzheimer's disease. Am J Psychiatry 1996;148:1159–63.
[17] Holroyd S, Currie LJ, Abraham IL. Aggression in a rural psychogeriatric outreach program. Int J Geriatr Psychiatry 1996;11:529–33.
[18] Morriss RK, Rovner BW, Folstein MF, et al. Delusions in newly admitted residents of nursing homes. Am J Psychiatry 1990;147:299–302.
[19] Heston LL, Gerrard J, Makris L. Inadequate treatment of depressed nursing home elderly. J Am Geriatr Soc 1992;40:117–22.
[20] Burns BJ, Wagner HR, Taube JE, et al. Mental health service use by the elderly in nursing homes. Am J Public Health 1993;83:331.
[21] Foster JR, Cataldo JK. Prediction of first episode of clinical depression in patients newly admitted to a medical long-term care facility: findings from a prospective study. Int J Geriatr Psychiatry 1993;8:297.
[22] Katz IR, Parmelee PA. Depression in elderly patients in residential care settings. In: Schneider LS, Reynolds III CF, Lebowitz BD, Freidhoff AJ, editors. Diagnosis and treatment of depression in late life. Washington, DC: American Psyciatric Press; 1994. p. 437.
[23] Katz IR, Lescher E, Kleban M. Clinical features of depression in the nursing home. Int Psychogeriatr 1989;1:5.
[24] Kafonek S, Ettinger WH, Roca R. Instruments for screening for depression and dementia in a long term care facility. J Am Geriatr Soc 1989;37:29.
[25] Rovner BW, German PS, Brant LJ. Depression and mortality in nursing homes. JAMA 1991; 265:993–6.
[26] Snowden J. Dementia, depression, and life satisfaction in nursing homes. Int J Geriatr Psychiatry 1986;1:85.
[27] Abrams RC, Teresi JA, Butin DN. Depression in nursing home residents. Clin Geriatr Med 1992; 8:309.
[28] Koenig HG, Blazer DDG. Epidemiology of geriatric affective disorders. Clin Geriatr Med 1992; 8:235.
[29] Parmelee PA, Katz IR, Lawton MP. Anxiety and its association with depression among institutionalized elderly. Am J Geriatr Psychiatry 1993;1:46.
[30] Cohen-Mansfield J, Marx MS, Werner P. Agitation in elderly persons: an integrative report of findings in a nursing home. Int Psychogeriatr 1992;4(Suppl 2):221.
[31] Cohen-Mansfield J, Werner P, Marx MS. Screaming in nursing home residents. J Am Geriatr Soc 1990;38:785.
[32] Parmelee PA, Katz IR, Lawton MP. The relation of pain to depression among institutionalized aged. J Gerontol 1991;46:P15.
[33] Cohen-Mansfield J, Marx MS. Pain and depression in the nursing home: corroborating results. J Gerontol 1993;48:P96.
[34] Borson S, McDonald GJ, Gayle T. Improvement in mood, physical symptoms and function with

nortriptyline for depression in patients with chronic obstructive pulmonary disease. Psychosomatics 1992;33:190.
[35] Katon W. Depression: relationship to somatization and chronic medical illness. J Clin Psychiatry 1984;45:4.
[36] Hsu LKJ, Zimmer B. Eating disorders in old age. Int J Eating Disord 1988;7:133.
[37] Miller DK, Morley JE, Rubenstein LZ, Pietruszka FM. Abnormal eating attitudes and body image in older undernourished individuals. J Am Geriatr Soc 1991;39:462.
[38] DeDeyn PP. Risperidone in the treatment of behavioral and psychological symptoms of dementia. Int J Psychogeriatr 2000;12(Suppl 1):263–9.
[39] Tune LE. Risperidone for the treatment of behavioral and psychological symptoms of dementia. J Clin Psychiatry 2001;62(Suppl 21):29–32.
[40] Wooltorton G. Risperidone (Risperdal): increased rate of cerebrovascular events in dementia trails. Canadian Medical Association 2003;167:1269.

ELSEVIER
SAUNDERS

Clin Geriatr Med 20 (2004) 93–119

CLINICS IN GERIATRIC MEDICINE

Cultural influences on dementia recognition and management

Jennifer J. Manly, PhD[a], David V. Espino, MD[b,*]

[a]Cognitive Neuroscience Division, GH Sergievsky Center and Taub Institute for Research on Alzheimer's Disease & The Aging Brain, Columbia University Health Science Center, 630 West 168th Street, P&S Box 16, New York, NY 10032, USA

[b]Department of Family & Community Medicine, University of Texas Health Science Center at San Antonio, 7703 Floyd Curl Drive, MC 7795, San Antonio, TX 78229-3900, USA

Changes in the ethnic and racial landscape among the elderly in the United States suggest that ethnic minority populations will bear an increased share of the economic and social burden associated with diseases that predominantly affect the elderly, such as Alzheimer's disease (AD) and other progressive dementias. The US Census Bureau estimates that the proportion of elders who are white and non-Hispanic will decline from 87% (in 1990) to 67% in 2050. By the year 2010, the population of Hispanic elders is expected to double and will be 11 times greater by 2050. Of the 80.1 million elderly projected for 2050, 8.4 million (10.4%) will be black, compared with 8% of elders in 1990.

Cross-cultural dementia research may provide an opportunity to identify elderly within the same ethnic group with different prevalence rates of AD that could enhance the search for risk factors [1]. Investigations of ethnic populations that have migrated across several cultures offer the opportunity to study groups for which genetic factors essentially remain the same but environmental and cultural forces undergo dramatic change. At the same time, comparison of different racial groups residing in the same environment with similar socioeconomic status and equal exposure to risk factors may help to uncover genetic factors responsible for AD.

The studies reviewed in this article examine ethnic differences in rates of broad categories, such as cognitive impairment or dementia, as well as specific neurodegenerative diseases, such as AD and vascular dementia. Cognitive

* Corresponding author.
E-mail address: espino@uthscsa.edu (D.V. Espino).

doi:10.1016/j.cger.2003.10.004

impairment, a necessary prerequisite for diagnosis of any dementia, is determined using either screening tests, such as the Mini-Mental State Exam (MMSE), or more sensitive and extensive neuropsychologic test batteries incorporating individual measures such as logical memory from the Wechsler Memory Scale. To meet clinical criteria for dementia, cognitive impairment must be of sufficient severity to interfere with activities of daily living. Cross-cultural research on dementia must contend with the fact that assessments of both cognitive impairment and daily functioning are susceptible to culturally dependent definitions and are quantified by measures that are sensitive to cultural and educational background.

There are many possible etiologies of progressive dementia, but the most frequent causes are Alzheimer's pathology and cerebrovascular disease. Although the exact etiology cannot be definitively determined before an autopsy, there are research criteria for AD and vascular dementia that have been shown to predict the specific pathologic determination upon autopsy with up to 90% accuracy. However, the supporting research has involved almost exclusively white subjects. Few autopsy studies have been performed to confirm the accuracy of these diagnoses among ethnic minorities.

This article reviews the impact of AD and dementia within four ethnic groups within the United States (African Americans, Hispanics, Asian/Pacific Islanders, and American Indians). It then explores some issues in the recognition of dementia among these populations, including cultural bias in measurement of cognitive functioning and differences in presentation of cognitively impaired elders across ethnic and cultural groups.

Impact of Alzheimer's disease and dementia across cultures

A number of studies have compared the rates of dementia and AD between ethnic groups residing in the United States. Despite differences in sampling methods and definitions of dementia as well as in definitions of race/ethnicity, the most frequent findings in reviewing this literature are that African Americans and Hispanics have higher prevalence and incidence of dementia and AD than whites. Native Americans appeared to have lower rates of AD in comparison to whites. Asian Americans had rates of dementia comparable to whites; however, whether there is the same proportion of AD compared with vascular dementia among Asian Americans and among Asian immigrants remains uncertain. Opinion differs on whether correction for education accounted for the different rates of dementia and AD found among these cultural groups.

Most United States-based studies have focused on comparing rates of dementia or AD among African Americans and Hispanics with rates among whites. These studies found higher rates of cognitive impairment, dementia, and AD among ethnic minorities than among whites [2]. One of the largest projects, a population-based, longitudinal study of 2126 elderly residents of the Washington Heights and Inwood communities of New York City, examined the incidence of AD among whites, African Americans, and Caribbean Hispanics [3]. Using National Institute of Neurological and Communicative Disorders and Stroke and the Alzheimer's Disease and Related Disorders Associations (NINCDS-ADRDA) criteria, neurologic examination, and results from an extensive neuropsychologic test, the standardized incidence rate for African American elders (4.2% per person-year) and Caribbean Hispanics (3.8% per person-year) was significantly higher than that of the referent group, non-Hispanic whites, even after correcting for differences in years of education.

Another large study, the Duke Established Populations for Epidemiological Studies of the Elderly (EPESE) project, found no differences in frequency of dementia between African Americans and whites. This study described a sample of 4136 participants, 55% of whom were black. The authors used the Consortium to Establish a Registry for Alzheimer's Disease (CERAD) Neuropsychological Test battery to assess cognitive functioning, and norms correcting for years of education [4] were used for the determination of significant cognitive deficit and dementia. The prevalence of dementia among elders above age 67, as determined by clinical consensus, was 7.0% for blacks and 7.2% for whites. There were also no differences in the 3-year incidence of dementia for blacks (5.8%) versus whites (6.2%). The investigators did not report incidence of dementia subtypes; therefore, it is possible that although the overall rates of dementia were similar among African Americans and whites, the frequencies of AD and vascular dementia may differ within the groups.

Hugh Hendrie and colleagues from the Indiana University School of Medicine and the University of Ibadan, Nigeria, are investigating the epidemiology of dementia among community-dwelling African Americans living in Indianapolis and Yoruba living in Ibadan. This study hoped to take advantage of the fact that African Americans are predominantly of the lineage of West African blacks but reside in quite different environments than Nigerians and are therefore likely to have different exposures to possible environmental risk factors. A total of 2212 African American elders and 2494 Nigerians were assessed [5]. Diagnoses were made under WHO guidelines, using DSM-II-R and ICD-10 criteria for dementia and NINCDS-ADRDA criteria for AD. Age-adjusted prevalence rates for dementia (2.29%) and AD (1.41%) among community-dwelling Yoruba elders in Ibadan were significantly lower than rates of dementia (8.24%) and AD (6.24%) among African Americans. Age-standardized annual incidence rates of dementia (1.35%) and AD (1.15%) are significantly lower in Ibadan than rates of dementia (3.24%) and AD (2.52%) among African Americans in Indiana [6]. Investigators in the Indianapolis-Ibadan study suggested several possible explanations for reduced rates among Nigerian elders, including differential mortality (those who would eventually develop AD may die at a younger age in Nigeria); the relatively younger age structure of the population; absence of environmental factors that might increase risk of AD; and disparate diagnostic criteria for functional decline. The investigators also suggested that the Nigerians may have a lower rate of amyloid deposition compared with African Americans.

The rate of dementia on admission to nursing homes is higher among black residents than among white residents [7]; however, findings from studies of long-term outcomes for African American elders with dementia are not consistent. Mortality associated with dementia was found to be higher among blacks than non-Hispanic whites, especially among black males [8]. However, there were no statistically significant differences in survival from time of entry into the CERAD study of whites and African Americans after accounting for the effects of age, gender, and severity of dementia [9].

The role of immigration and changes in environmental risk factors were examined in several epidemiologic studies of elders with Japanese ancestry. The age-standardized prevalence of dementia (using DSM-III criteria) among Japanese American men aged 71 to 93 years living in Hawaii [10] was 7.6%. This was higher than Japanese men living in Japan (4% to 6%), similar to European populations. The age-standardized prevalence of AD (using NINCDS-ADRDA criteria) in this Japanese American population was 4.7%. The investigators suggested that environmental or cultural exposures associated with migration from Japan to Hawaii influenced the development of AD in these Japanese Americans. Similar results were reported in a study of 1985 Japanese American participants in the *Kame* project in King County, Washington [11]. A cross-sectional study of dementia prevalence using the California Alzheimer's Disease and Diagnostic Treatment Centers found that compared with whites, Asian Americans had a greater proportion of vascular dementia and lower proportion of AD [12], similar to studies of Asians in Asia.

It appears that Native Americans have a lower rate of AD than whites but equivalent rates of overall cognitive impairment or dementia. Hendrie et al [13] examined 192 Cree living on two reserves in Manitoba, Canada, aged 65 and over, and an age-stratified sample of 241 English-speaking whites living in Winnipeg. Using the Community Screening Interview for Dementia (CSI-D) to screen for cognitive impairment, the researchers found a significant difference between the age-adjusted prevalence of AD among the Cree Indians (0.5%) as compared with whites (3.5%), despite the two groups having an equivalent age-adjusted prevalence of dementia (4.2% in each population).

A study of Cherokee Indians living in northeastern Oklahoma [14] used NINCDS-ADRDA criteria to identify 26 people aged 65 years and older with AD and then assessed an equal number of normal controls. The investigators found that as the genetic degree of Cherokee ancestry increased, the frequency of AD decreased. That is, independent of APOE $\varepsilon 4$ allele status, elders with more than 50% genetic Cherokee ancestry were less likely to be in the AD group than the control group. Genetic degree of ancestry for each participant was calculated using genealogic records provided by the Cherokee Nation Tribal Registration Department. A limitation of this study is its case-control design; however, this study represents a more advanced method of examining the relationship of race/ethnicity to disease because the degree of ethnic ancestry was assessed (albeit not through formal genetic analysis), as opposed to classifying individuals into racial groups based on self-report or investigator observation.

Autopsy confirmation of Alzheimer's disease pathology

Neuropathologic confirmation of the presence and severity of AD pathology among patients diagnosed with AD is the only way to confirm ethnic discrepancies in AD prevalence and incidence. However, African Americans and other ethnic minorities are less likely to consent to autopsy [15–17]. Therefore, there are few published studies comparing the rates of neuropathologically defined AD among different ethnic groups in the United States; most published neuropathologic studies of AD have examined whites almost exclusively. The few studies with ethnically diverse samples have found, among those autopsied, no racial differences in frequency of AD pathology [18] or that AD lesions are more prevalent among whites than among blacks [19]. Small sample size is a problem for each of these studies, and because there is a much lower rate of consent for autopsy among African Americans, there may be a selection bias.

One study avoided selection bias by performing a survey of all autopsies on individuals age 40 to 70 in the Maryland Chief Medical Examiner's office for an 8-year period [20]. All died of "non-natural" causes, mostly accidents and homicides. The researchers assessed the prevalence of senile plaques (SP) and neurofibrillary tangles (NFT) in three brain areas: the hippocampus, entorhinal cortex, and the inferior temporal cortex. In their sample of 138 individuals, 42% were African American and 61% were younger than age 65. NFTs were most common after age 54 and were found mostly in hippocampus and entorhinal cortex. SPs were less frequent overall but were found mostly in people 75 years and older in the entorhinal cortex and inferior temporal cortex. Prevalence of neuritic plaques was consistently lower in African Americans than among whites. Although the researchers confirmed that prevalence of mixed SP and NFT was strongly correlated with age, there was no evidence that these pathologic changes had any differences in frequency by race.

Imaging evidence

Brain imaging studies, using both structural and functional methods, might provide an alternative line of evidence concerning AD pathology that could back up the epidemiologic findings of ethnic discrepancies in AD. However, there are very few studies of structural or functional brain imaging using diverse groups of elders. Studies of African American elders with clinical diagnoses of AD have shown that magnetic resonance imaging (MRI)-determined measurements of hippocampal volume [21] and qualitative computed tomography (CT) and MRI findings [22] were similar to those reported in other imaging studies of primarily white patients. One study using MRI and single photon emission CT (SPECT) showed no major ethnic differences in degree of white matter hyperintensities (WMH), ventricle-to-brain ratio (VBR), and uptake among 3301 nondemented community-dwelling elders without a history of stroke or transient ischemic attack [23]. Other research has found a higher prevalence of white matter lesions among nondemented African Americans elders, a predictable finding given that cardiovascular risk factors (eg, hypertension, diabetes) are more common among African Americans [24,25].

Instrumentation issues in detection of dementia across cultures

Ethnic differences and cognitive testing

Research criteria for dementia [26] and probable or possible AD [27] require documentation of memory and other cognitive impairment through neuropsychologic testing. However, few cognitive ability measures have been properly validated for use among ethnic minorities in the United States. Lack of such validation may account for the fact that, based on neuropsychologic test performance, ethnic minorities are judged to be cognitively impaired more often than non-Hispanic white people. This section reviews studies within and outside the United States that have compared the cognitive test performance of different ethnic groups and describe constructs that might allow for more sophisticated investigations of ethnic differences in the future.

Use of the standard cut-off of 23 on the MMSE leads to overdiagnosis of dementia among African Americans, even after controlling for years of education [28]. Racial, ethnic, and cultural differences have been found on MMSE performance and other screening measures before [4,29] and after adjusting for education [30–35].

Difficulties in interpreting cognitive scores among ethnic minority elders are not limited to brief screening instruments; several studies have indicated that ethnic or cultural factors have a substantial effect on neuropsychologic batteries [36,37]. Even when ethnic groups are matched on socioeconomic variables, discrepancies in neuropsychologic test performance have remained [38–41]. Roberts and Hamsher [42] found that neurologically intact whites obtained significantly higher scores on a measure of visual naming ability than did neurologically intact African Americans, even after correcting for education level. Several other studies also reported ethnic differences in performance on tests of visual confrontation naming [33,43,44].

Ethnicity-related differences have been reported on measures of nonverbal abilities as well [45–49]. Jacobs et al [38] found that Spanish-speaking elders scored significantly lower than age- and education-matched English-speaking elders on a measure of nonverbal abstraction (ie, the Identities and Oddities subtest from the Mattis Dementia Rating Scale); multiple choice matching and recognition formats of the Benton Visual Retention Test; and measures of category fluency and comprehension. In another study, healthy Spanish-speaking Mexicans and Mexican Americans who lived near a United States–Mexico border (n = 200) were compared with residents of Madrid, Spain (n = 218). After accounting for education, borderland residents obtained significantly lower scores on measures of recognition discriminability for stories and figures, learned fewer details from a story over five trials, and made more perseverative responses on the Wisconsin Card Sorting Task [50]. There were some interactions between years of education and place of birth, suggesting that among those with high levels of education, borderland and Spanish participants performed similarly on several measures.

Several studies have reported significant differences in performance on neuropsychologic test batteries designed to detect dementia among African American and white elders despite correcting for years of education, age, occupational attainment, or history of medical conditions such as hypertension and diabetes [4,40,51]. In contrast, a number of studies have failed to find discrepancies in test performance between racial, ethnic, or cultural groups after participants were matched on years of education [44,52], after statistically adjusting for education [53–55], or after cut-off scores were adjusted for those with low education [56]. However, the statistical power to detect a significant difference in some of these studies was severely limited by their small sample sizes of non-white participants. For example, there were no significant ethnic differences among a small number of African Americans (n = 11) and whites (n = 32) with AD on measures of naming, picture vocabulary, verbal abstraction, verbal list learning, and pragmatic language use after controlling for MMSE score and years of education [57]. Another study found that among 18 black and 114 white participants who met NINCDS-ADRDA criteria for AD, there were no significant differences by race on decline in MMSE score over an average 2.5-year period, whereas left-handedness, more years of education, and family history of dementia were associated with more rapid decline [58].

Taken together, most previous studies of ethnic group differences in performance on the MMSE and neuropsychologic tests have shown that discrepancies between scores of different ethnic groups persist, despite equating groups on other demographics such as age, education, gender, and socioeconomic background. These discrepancies cause attenuated specificity of verbal and nonverbal neuropsychologic tests, such that cognitively normal ethnic minorities are more likely to be misdiagnosed as impaired as compared with whites [33,40,59–61]. These findings indicate that not all tasks are functionally equivalent [62,63]. Although establishing separate test norms for ethnic minorities may help with misdiagnosis [64], variability of educational and cultural experiences within ethnicity may decrease the accuracy of these norms. Separate norms do not address the variables related to culture, race, and education that underlie ethnic group differences on cognitive test performance. It is possible that separate ethnic group norms will create more problems than they solve, lead to increased misunderstanding of racial and ethnic group differences, and become unwieldy to the everyday practitioner. Instead, direct measurement of more meaningful and predictive variables that underlie test performance across cultural groups may serve to increase accuracy of cognitive assessment and increase the validity of all instruments used to diagnose dementia. In the next sections, we review the relationship of some of the variables that differ within and between racial and ethnic groups to cognitive test performance.

Acculturation

Most previous research on ethnicity has classified participants on the basis of physical appearance or self-identified racial/ethnic classification rather than measuring the cultural variables that accompany ethnic group membership. However, as suggested by Helms [62], specification of experiential, attitudinal, or behavioral variables that distinguish those belonging to different ethnic groups, and also vary among individuals within an ethnic group, may allow investigators to understand better the underlying reasons for the relationship between ethnic background and cognitive test performance.

Level of acculturation is one way in which social scientists have operationalized within-group cultural variability. Acculturation is defined as the level at which people participate in the values, language, and practices of their own ethnic community versus those of the dominant culture [65,66]. Previous studies have identified ideologies, beliefs, expectations, and attitudes as important components of acculturation, as well as cognitive and behavioral characteristics such as language and customs [65,67–69].

Few studies have examined the relationship of cognitive test performance to within-group ethnic or cultural factors independent of those associated with socioeconomic status. Arnold et al [70] found a relationship between Hispanic acculturation and performance on selected tests of the Halstead-Reitan Battery among college students. Artiola et al [50] reported that among Mexican and Mexican American residents of a United States border region, the percentage of time in which individuals lived in the United States was significantly and negatively related to number of words generated on a Spanish oral fluency measure, especially among those with fewer than 8 years of education. In addition, those who spent a larger percentage of their life in the United States made more perseverative errors on the Wisconsin Card Sorting Test, and bilingualism accounted for a significant amount of variance in performance on a Spanish Verbal Learning Test [50].

Three studies have explored the relationship of African-American acculturation (as measured by the African American Acculturation Scale [71,72]) to cognitive test performance. Manly et al [73] found that among neurologically intact African Americans between the ages of 20 and 65, those who were less acculturated (more traditional) obtained lower scores on measures of general information and naming than more acculturated African Americans. Among elderly residents of northern Manhattan [74], acculturation accounted for a significant amount of variance in several neuropsychologic measures assessing verbal and nonverbal abilities after accounting for age, education, and gender. Among elderly African Americans living in Jacksonville, Florida, acculturation accounted for a significant amount of variance in verbal intelligence quotient (IQ, as measured by the Wechsler Adult Intelligence Scale), Boston Naming Test, and delayed recall of stories from the Wechsler Memory Scale–Revised [75].

Taken together, investigations of acculturation level suggest that there are cultural differences within elders of the same ethnicity that relate to neuropsychologic measures of verbal and nonverbal skills, and that accounting for acculturation may improve the accuracy of certain neuropsychologic tests. Although previous research has focused on ethnic minority elders in the United States, it is likely that within-group cultural differences are also significant factors in the test performance of American elders who identify themselves as white, as well as ethnic groups outside the United States.

Years of education, quality of education, and literacy

Extreme differences in educational levels are often found between ethnic minorities and whites. Illiteracy rates in the United States are highest among people aged 65 and over but are especially elevated among ethnic minority elders [76]. Cross-cultural researchers are therefore challenged to find measures sensitive to cognitive impairment across these broad educational backgrounds [63]. Although it is common for investigators to use covariance, matching procedures, or education-corrected norms to "equate" ethnic groups on years of education before interpreting neuropsychologic test performance, as discussed previously, these techniques ignore ethnic discrepancies in quality of education. Therefore, disparate school experiences could explain why many ethnic minorities obtain lower scores on cognitive measures even after controlling for years of education.

Therefore, support of ethnic and racial group differences depends on whether we can successfully "adjust" for years of education. However, along with several other researchers [77–79], we argue that due to the disparities in quality of education, matching on quantity of formal education does not necessarily mean that the quality of education received by each racial group is comparable. The variable "years of education" systematically differs between African Americans and whites [80–85] and is also related to cognitive test performance. If this variable is not commensurate between racial groups, residual confounding will occur and spurious racial differences will be interpreted despite matching groups on years of education.

Presence of poor literacy skills among elders is also a particularly relevant issue for neuropsychologists attempting to accurately detect dementia using cognitive measures. Reading level is a very powerful predictor of cognitive test performance, independent of years of education, age, or ethnicity [86–93]. These results suggest that interpretation of performance on verbal and nonverbal cognitive measures is more dependent on knowledge of literacy or reading skills than years of education.

Our group recently reported a study that sought to determine if discrepancies in quality of education could explain differences in cognitive test score between African American and white elders matched on years of education [94]. A comprehensive neuropsychologic battery was administered to a sample of nondemented African American and non-Hispanic white participants in an epidemiologic study of normal aging and dementia in the northern Manhattan community. The Reading Recognition subtest from the Wide Range Achievement Test-version 3 (WRAT-3) was used as an estimate of quality of education. African

American elders obtained significantly lower scores than whites on measures of word list learning and memory, figure memory, abstract reasoning, fluency, and visuospatial skill even though the groups were matched on years of education. However, after adjusting for the WRAT-3 reading score, the overall effect of race was greatly reduced, and racial differences on all tests (except category fluency and a drawing measure) became nonsignificant. Reading score also attenuated the effect of race after accounting for an estimate of test-wiseness. This finding suggests that years of education is an inadequate measure of the educational experience among multicultural elders, and that adjusting for quality of education may improve the specificity of certain neuropsychologic measures across racial groups.

These findings suggest that the full extent of discrepancies in educational experience between African Americans and whites are not captured by a simple "highest grade attained" variable, and thus residual confounding may explain findings of "persistent" race effects after matching groups on years of education. Nevertheless, despite the clear improvement in specificity that is provided by adjusting cognitive test scores for differences in educational experience across ethnic groups, some researchers caution against controlling for educational variables in studies of dementia, as low education may itself be a risk factor for disease.

Low education has been established as a significant risk factor for AD and other dementias [95]. A higher prevalence of AD and dementia among elders with low levels of education has been found in Brazil [96], China [97,98], Finland [99], France [100], Italy [101,102], Israel [103,104], the Netherlands [105], Sweden [106,107], and the United States [108–110]. Higher incidence of dementia has been demonstrated in several studies [111–114]. Cognitive decline appears to be faster [115–117] and associated with increased risk of mortality [118] among highly educated minorities with AD, which suggests that the level of brain pathology is greater by the time well-educated individuals show the signs of dementia.

The studies reviewed in the previous section focus on the relationship of schooling and literacy to dementia or AD. But there is also evidence for a role of education in age-related cognitive decline. Several studies of normal aging have reported more rapid cognitive and functional decline among individuals with lower educational attainment [119–125]. These studies suggest that the same education-related factors that delay the onset of dementia also allow individuals to cope more effectively with changes encountered in normal aging.

Cognitive reserve has been suggested as the mechanism for the link between low education and higher risk of dementia and cognitive decline observed in these studies [126–128]. Reserve, or the brain's ability to tolerate the effects of dementia pathology, may result from native ability or from the effects of lifetime experience. Years of education may serve as a proxy for reserve whether it results from ability or experience. In passive models of reserve [126], education would be a proxy for the brain's capacity (synaptic density or complexity) to tolerate either gradual or sudden insult. In active models, years of education would be an indicator of the brain's ability to compensate for pathology through more efficient use of existing cognitive networks or recruitment of alternate networks.

However, there are cases in which the relationship between education and risk for cognitive impairment or dementia is weakened or absent. Two large international studies of incident dementia found that illiteracy or low levels of education did not increase the risk of AD among elders in India [129] and West Africa [130,131]. In fact, these studies had the lowest prevalence and incidence rates of dementia observed to date despite the fact that a large proportion of the populations lacked formal schooling or literacy training. This paradox serves to illuminate the difficulty in comparing cultural groups with disparate backgrounds. Reserve is measured by proxy variables (such as years of education, occupational level, or IQ measures), but there are a number of ways in which cultural, racial, and economic factors may affect the predictive power of these proxies. First, it is possible that race- and income-based limits on educational opportunity weaken the relationship between years of education and native ability, leading to underestimates of the relationship between education and cognitive decline. Minorities with strong intellectual abilities may not achieve high levels of academic or occupational status because their opportunities are limited by societal forces (eg, racism, poverty) unrelated to their native intellect or drive to succeed. Although such individuals may be powerful or influential in their community, their abilities may not be reflected in years of schooling or traditional indicators of occupational status. Alternatively, rather than a reflection of innate ability, years of education could be an indicator of lifetime experiences that change the brain during childhood or adult life and thus create a reserve against disease pathology. However, use of years of education to represent a direct effect of experience on the brain or cognition is also problematic for ethnic minorities and immigrants due to the increased discordance between years of education and quality of education among these groups.

We propose that literacy could be a more sensitive proxy for reserve than years of education, because it more accurately reflects the quality of the educational experience provided to ethnic minority elders. In addition, literacy could be a more accurate reflection of native ability because it does not assume that all individuals get the same amount of learning from a certain grade level; the fact that some excel more than others or seek learning outside of school will be reflected in measurements of literacy.

We designed a study to explore the relationship of literacy level to change in memory ability over time among an ethnically diverse sample of English-speaking nondemented elders [132]. Specifically, we wanted to determine if literacy was a stronger predictor of memory decline (and thus a more sensitive indicator of reserve) than years of education or racial/ethnic classification, although each of these variables were expected to influence baseline scores. We focused our analyses on immediate and delayed recall measures from a verbal word list learning task, because these measures are sensitive to age-related memory decline and the earliest signs of AD. Among 136 participants, we found that elders with both high and low levels of literacy declined in immediate and delayed memory over time; however, the decline was more rapid among low literacy elders. This suggests that high literacy skills do not provide complete preservation of memory skills but rather a slowing of age-related decline. All participants had normal overall cognition and were functioning normally in daily activities; thus, the decline in memory scores was not associated with the onset of a dementia disorder. There were no interactions between time and either years of education or ethnicity, suggesting that in this diverse population of normal elders, literacy was the most sensitive predictor of memory decline. Unlike many previous studies that examined the relationship of education to dementia or normal aging, we did not find that low education (< 12 years) was a risk factor for cognitive decline.

Racial socialization

Level of comfort and confidence during the testing session may also vary among ethnic minorities. The concept of stereotype threat has been described as a factor that may attenuate the performance of racial minorities on cognitive tests. Stereotype threat describes the effect of attention diverting from the task at hand to the concern that one's performance will confirm a negative stereotype about one's group. When a test consisting of difficult verbal GRE exam items was described as measuring intellectual ability, black undergraduates at Stanford University performed worse than SAT score-matched whites [133,134]. However, when the same test was described as a "laboratory problem-solving task" or a "challenging test" unrelated to intellectual ability, scores of African Americans matched those of white students. Researchers have also shown that when gender differences in math ability were invoked, stereotype threat undermined performance of women on math tests [135], and among white males (when comparisons with Asians were invoked) [136]. The role of stereotype threat in neuropsychologic test performance of African Americans and Hispanics has not been investigated. It is likely that the salience of negative stereotypes differs among racial minorities, and therefore, stereotype threat will likely affect some test takers more than others. Investigation of the experiential, social, and cultural variables that affect vulnerability to stereotype threat should be examined.

Linguistic issues

Translation of English-language tests

Clinicians and researchers sometimes erroneously assume that instruments are equivalent across populations as long as the test is administered in the native language of the individual. However, literal translation may not produce items with comparable word frequency or salience in each culture, resulting in different difficulty levels [79,137,138]. In addition, idiosyncrasies of different languages may introduce problems in equating certain tests. For example, when asked to name as many animals as possible in a minute, Hispanics produce fewer exemplars than do Vietnamese. This discrepancy can be explained by the fact that most animal names in Spanish are multisyllabic, whereas most animal names in Vietnamese are monosyllabic [139].

Translators of cognitive measures must use extreme caution and proper methods to adapt measures into another language. Artiola and colleagues [140] describe several examples of Spanish versions of tests that include syntactic, lexical, and spelling errors. These authors also suggest that investigators consult only those who possess native fluency and in-depth knowledge of the culture before attempting to translate a measure. The accuracy of translated and adapted instruments should be checked following established guidelines [79,140–143]. Researchers and clinicians must also develop standards to determine in which language bilinguals should be assessed [144].

Translation of measures is not simply a linguistic issue; measures must be culturally equivalent as well. It must be determined whether the use of a particular test format to assess the cognitive skill of interest is equally valid within every culture in which the test will be administered [137,145].

Norms

Investigators must be aware that the published norms for tests administered in English are not necessarily valid when the tests are administered in another language. Further, they should not assume that test norms can be applied to distinct populations simply because they share a language. For example, there is evidence that several instruments developed in Spanish-speaking countries may not be functionally or linguistically equivalent when used among Spanish speakers in the United States [50]. Similarly, tests and norms developed among a particular group of immigrants to the United States (eg, Cuban Americans) may not be valid among other groups in the United States who share a language (eg, Dominicans or Puerto Ricans) [79].

Diagnostic and management considerations

Language

Certain characteristics among the elderly minority populations may hinder health professionals in the diagnosis and treatment of dementia. One characteristic is that of language. Mutchler and Brallier [146] found that one third of elder Hispanics lacks English proficiency and are "linguistically isolated." Elder Asian American or Arab Americans also commonly are unable to communicate clearly with the health care provider. Yano found that language of interview impacted on cognitive status testing in elder Japanese Americans with those being tested in the language that they were most comfortable with doing best [147]. A recent review concluded that although it has been argued that cognitive status assessment instruments are culturally biased, the available published evidence suggests that the fundamental issue is the elders' language ability, rather than minority group membership [148]. Misinterpretation is a serious threat to the reliability and validity of testing. Family members are often used as translators but are not likely to be objective or familiar with medical terminology. And even translators who are reasonably fluent in both languages may not be familiar with many of the terms used in neuropsychologic testing [149,150]. Increasing the linguistic diversity of testers and improving the availability of objective translators are thus worthwhile goals for investigators; when this is not feasible, the possibility of misinterpretation must be taken into consideration when interpreting results.

Therefore, the inability of the health care provider to accurately ascertain information using standard health screening questions or through more objective neuropsychologic testing will incorrectly lead the provider to both misdiagnose and mismanage monolingual minority elders early in their dementing illness. As mentioned, the language problem is compounded when untrained translators are used. Bilingual staff, who are frequently called on to serve as translators, are often ill prepared to deal with the complexities of the dementia evaluation and ongoing care. These translator staff members may have variable English skills as well. This may lead to problems of interpreter-patient interactions, poor paraphrasing, and bias in reporting due to interpreter ethnocentric beliefs concerning physical and mental health and poorer patient satisfaction [151]. Providers should be attentive in providing formal translation services. Formal translation services such as those provided by AT&T have resulted in enhanced patient satisfaction [152].

Socioeconomic status

The lack of formal education among minority elderly may compound health care provider-patient communication problems when mental status is being evaluated. It has been estimated that only 43.7% of blacks and 29.4% of Hispanics have a high school diploma compared with 71.6% of elder non-Hispanic whites [153]. Standard written or verbal questions and phrases that are used by health professionals to assess health status may be at a level of sophistication that elicits inaccurate responses from elderly African Americans or Hispanics, both during diagnosis and during ongoing treatment.

Financial issues can present a major burden for minority families and their loved ones with a dementing illness. Blacks are less likely than whites to have supplemental Medicare insurance [154]. Furthermore, elderly minorities are more likely to skip medication doses or otherwise avoid using their prescription medications because of cost [155]. Senior health maintenance organizations do increase access to health services for minority elders but at the cost of lower satisfaction [156]. Therefore, decisions that minority families make regarding the care of their loved one with dementia incorporate finances to a great degree. Providers should be alert to decreasing this burden through identification of governmental or community-based dementia care resources.

Transportation and neighborhood

Transportation becomes a major issue in highly urbanized areas. Regardless of financial status, the rendering of a minority elder as not able to drive creates additional burdens on the caregiving unit but becomes a major issue for elder minorities with limited resources. The location of a hospital, clinic, or pharmacy may yield it inaccessible to older minorities [157,158]. Inpatient or ambulatory facilities within the minority community that don't afford easy access by elderly residents and their families will not be used by these individuals. Additionally, inadequate planning and resources to meet the transportation needs of the older minorities will render such facilities ineffective [159].

Additionally, recent findings that barrio residents have almost three times greater risk for cognitive dysfunction than those Mexican American elders living elsewhere suggest that where a cognitively impaired elder lives makes a difference [160]. Those living in lower income neighborhoods may be in need of more dementia diagnostic and treatment services, yet be unable to access them.

Provider–patient relationship

Minority elders most likely present to the provider for diagnosis at higher levels of cognitive impairment and with other psychiatric symptoms that require the provider's additional time and attention [161,162]. Furthermore, good provider–patient relationships are essential in dealing with the family issues and complex decision making that occurs in the management of a minority elder with a dementing illness. Families and patients must feel that they are receiving the very best care. However, evidence suggests that providers may allow for less minority participation in the development of therapeutic plans than they do for white patients [163]. This participation may be a result of language barriers, trust issues, and failure to understand cultural contexts.

Language has been mentioned earlier in the context of diagnosis but remains intertwined with the doctor–patient relationship and is a significant barrier to health care services. It has been suggested that health care costs may be increased in non-English speaking patients as studies may be substituted for doctor–patient dialog [164,165]. Providers who care for large numbers of monolingual elders must be prepared to provide adequate translation services and be familiar with their use.

Also, established primary health care providers enjoy high levels of patient trust within their community. Minority patients may be less likely to trust their physician than nonminority patients [166,167]. Trust must be earned from both the minority patient and family if therapeutic relationships are to be established and effective dementia care rendered. Respect remains a significant unrecognized factor in minority populations.

Finally, providers should understand the primary cultural constructs of the primary minority populations that they serve. For example, the primary advance directive decision maker for the demented elder may be a family member rather than the elder themselves [168]. Indirect communication is common in both Asian and American Indian cultures [169]. Polite conversation is sometimes necessary to maintain good relations with both the minority family and patient [170]. The minority family or elder may prefer to have "everything done" in deference to the majority view of encouraging do-not-resuscitate status at an early dementia stage [171,172]. The provider should be culturally aware as minorities may be reluctant to discuss these issues openly.

Family support

In the United States, family caregiving remains the cornerstone of support for all elders with dementia. Although familism may be stronger in minority groups, the response of the family unit to the needs of the demented elder may result in higher levels of caregiver stress and burden [173,174]. Dilworth-Anderson and Gibson [175] found that among minorities with dementia, family caregiving processes and help-seeking behavior are influenced by how family members assign meaning to the dementing process. Thus, informing the extended minority family of the treatment alternatives and training family members to adapt to the behavioral changes that accompany a dementing illness may prevent the deterioration of the patients and caregivers. Long-term care placement of a minority demented elder may not be a viable option for the family unit or may require significant discussion by a large group of family members before institutionalization. Finally, care for the extended family unit, and the direct care provider in particular, will provide more direct care options for the demented minority elder over the long term. The increased reliance on family for an older member's care may place an economic and social strain on Hispanic families attempting to improve their socioeconomic status [176]. Such a strain may lead to a deterioration in the family dynamics that support the elder's health. It is beneficial for the health of elders if their guardians have the necessary information and assistance that will result in the family's participation with the health care plan. Minority families may be particularly receptive to this approach since they have traditionally assumed responsibility for the complete care of their aged family members.

Long-term care

The growing number of people progressing through the dementia stages has increased demand for nursing home accommodations. Minority families most likely view the nursing home as a "choice of last resort" with high levels of stress introduced into the family unit with the decision to institutionalize a demented elder [177,178]. This is constent with Weintraub and colleagues [179] who found that more African Americans with more severe levels of cognitive impairment than non-Hispanic whites were admitted to Wisconsin nursing homes. Wallace and colleagues [180] found that older African Americans are less likely to use nursing homes than whites, with the lower institutionalization replaced by a higher use of paid home care, informal-only care, and no care. It has been predicted that blacks and Hispanic nursing home admissions will continue to be less than that of non-Hispanic whites in the future [181].

Older minority groups tend to underuse long-term care services [180]. The primary reasons why minority groups may not use nursing homes include high cost, cultural custom insensitivity, disrespect, and abuse/neglect issues that are not uncommon to long-term care institutions. Huber and colleagues [182] found in examining a six-state ombudsman database that, while a larger percentage of racial minority complaints were verified, a lower percentage were resolved with the most common complaints being loss of dignity/respect, physical abuse, and gross neglect. Bernabei and colleagues [183] found that minority patients residing in nursing homes were also less likely than whites to have pain recorded even after adjustment for language differences with the trend noted for African Americans, Hispanics, Asians, and American Indians. Similar problems may play a role in the underuse of other long-term care services by elderly minorities with dementia. In general, outpatient health care facilities that serve a significant number of minority patients do not adequately address the cultural and language obstacles that their patients face [184]. Additional long-term care services, such as,bilingual caretakers, minority counselors, and case managers, would greatly benefit minorities with dementia and the families that care for them.

End-of-life issues

As the minority elder reaches the end stages of the dementing illness, care at the end of life is key to a successful management outcome. Minorities may continue to encounter significant barriers at this stage. Krakauer and colleagues [185] show that, in addition to the usual barriers to end-of-life care, minorities must deal with insensitivity to cultural differences in attitudes toward death and end-of-life care and issues related to mistrust of the health care system due to the history of racism in medicine. For example, Carrese and Rhodes [186] reported that exposing older Navajos to advanced care planning as required by the Patient Self-determination Act and the principle of autonomy can inadvertently harm them. Blackhall et al [187] found that Korean Americans and Mexican Americans were more likely than African Americans or European Americans to believe that only the family, and not the patient, should be told the truth about a diagnosis of metastatic cancer or a terminal prognosis and that the family rather than the patient should make decisions about life support. The terminal diagnosis may be shared first and only with the family in Japanese culture [188]. These cultural norms may extend across socioeconomic or educational lines [189]. Therefore, in dealing with minority patients, care providers must be sensitive to a family-centered style of information sharing that may directly conflict with their training in adherence to the patient autonomy model. Attention to cultural beliefs and practices of the populations providers serve, and inquiring whether an individual patient adheres to these cultural beliefs, will enable the provider to provide comprehensive and compassionate palliative care at the end of life [190].

Summary

More and more information is emerging on the prevalence and incidence of dementia in older minority groups. The development of more sophisticated instrumentation to assist the health care provider is ongoing. Minority groups have special issues that are unique from the general population with regard to diagnostic and management approaches. Health care providers of large groups of minority demented patients should be familiar with the particular needs of the groups they serve.

Acknowledgment

The authors would like to thank E. Mikaila Adams for the technical preparation of this book.

References

[1] Osuntokun BO, Hendrie HC, Ogunniyi AO, Hall KS, Lakwauwa UG, Brittain HM, et al. Cross-cultural studies in Alzheimer's disease. Ethn Dis 1992;2(4):352–7.

[2] Prineas RJ, Demirovic J, Bean JA, Duara R, Gomez-Martin O, Loewenstein DA, et al. South Florida Program on Aging and Health. Assessing the prevalence of Alzheimer's disease in three ethnic groups. J Fla Med Assoc 1995;82(12):805–10.

[3] Tang MX, Cross P, Andrews H, Jacobs DM, Small S, Bell K, et al. Incidence of AD in African-Americans, Caribbean Hispanics, and Caucasians in northern Manhattan. Neurology 2001; 56(1):49–56.

[4] Unverzagt FW, Hall KS, Torke AM, Rediger JD. Effects of age, education and gender on CERAD neuropsychological test performance in an African American sample. Clin Neuropsychol 1996;10:180–90.

[5] Hendrie HC, Osuntokun BO, Hall KS, Ogunniyi AO, Hui SL, Unverzagt FW, et al. Prevalence of Alzheimer's disease and dementia in two communities: Nigerian Africans and African Americans. Am J Psychiatr 1995;152(10):1485–92.

[6] Hendrie HC, Ogunniyi A, Hall KS, Baiyewu O, Unverzagt FW, Gureje O, et al. Incidence of dementia and Alzheimer disease in 2 communities: Yoruba residing in Ibadan, Nigeria, and African Americans residing in Indianapolis, Indiana. JAMA 2001;285(6):739–47.

[7] Weintraub D, Raskin A, Ruskin PE, Gruber-Baldini AL, Zimmerman SI, Hebel JR, et al. Racial differences in the prevalence of dementia among patients admitted to nursing homes. Psychiatr Serv 2000;51(10):1259–64.

[8] Lanska DJ. Dementia mortality in the United States. Results of the 1986 National Mortality Followback Survey. Neurology 1998;50(2):362–7.

[9] Heyman A, Peterson B, Fillenbaum G, Pieper C. The consortium to establish a registry for Alzheimer's disease (CERAD). Part XIV: demographic and clinical predictors of survival in patients with Alzheimer's disease. Neurology 1996;46(3):656–60.

[10] White L, Petrovitch H, Ross GW, Masaki KH, Abbott RD, Teng EL, et al. Prevalence of dementia in older Japanese-American men in Hawaii: the Honolulu-Asia Aging Study. JAMA 1996;276(12):955–60.

[11] Graves AB, Larson EB, Edland SD, Bowen JD, McCormick WC, McCurry SM, et al. Prevalence of dementia and its subtypes in the Japanese American population of King County, Washington state. The Kame Project. Am J Epidemiol 1996;144(8):760–71.

[12] Yeo G, Gallagher-Thompson D, Lieberman M. Variations in dementia characteristics by ethnic

category. In: Yeo G, Gallagher-Thompson D, editors. Ethnicity and the dementias. Washington, DC: Taylor and Francis; 1996. p. 21–30.
[13] Hendrie HC, Hall KS, Pillay N, Rodgers D, Prince C, Norton J, et al. Alzheimer's disease is rare in Cree. Int Psychogeriatr 1993;5(1):5–14.
[14] Rosenberg RN, Richter RW, Risser RC, Taubman K, Prado-Farmer I, Ebalo E, et al. Genetic factors for the development of Alzheimer disease in the Cherokee Indian. Arch Neurol 1996; 53(10):997–1000.
[15] Harrell LE, Callaway R, Powers R. Autopsy in dementing illness: who participates? Alzheimer Dis Assoc Disord 1993;7(2):80–7.
[16] Fillenbaum GG, Huber MS, Beekly D, Henderson VW, Mortimer J, Morris JC, et al. The consortium to establish a registry for Alzheimer's Disease (CERAD). Part XIII. Obtaining autopsy in Alzheimer's disease. Neurology 1996;46(1):142–5.
[17] Bonner GJ, Darkwa OK, Gorelick PB. Autopsy recruitment program for African Americans. Alzheimer Dis Assoc Disord 2000;14(4):202–8.
[18] Miller FD, Hicks SP, D'Amato CJ, Landis JR. A descriptive study of neuritic plaques and neurofibrillary tangles in an autopsy population. Am J Epidemiol 1984;120(3):331–41.
[19] de la Monte SM, Hutchins GM, Moore GW. Racial differences in the etiology of dementia and frequency of Alzheimer lesions in the brain. J Natl Med Assoc 1989;81(6):644–52.
[20] Sandberg G, Stewart W, Smialek J, Troncoso JC. The prevalence of the neuropathological lesions of Alzheimer's disease is independent of race and gender. Neurobiol Aging 2001; 22(2):169–75.
[21] Sencakova D, Graff-Radford NR, Willis FB, Lucas JA, Parfitt F, Cha RH, et al. Hippocampal atrophy correlates with clinical features of Alzheimer disease in African Americans. Arch Neurol 2001;58(10):1593–7.
[22] Charletta D, Gorelick PB, Dollear TJ, Freels S, Harris Y. CT and MRI findings among African-Americans with Alzheimer's disease, vascular dementia, and stroke without dementia. Neurology 1995;45(8):1456–61.
[23] Longstreth Jr WT, Arnold AM, Manolio TA, Burke GL, Bryan N, Jungreis CA, et al. Clinical correlates of ventricular and sulcal size on cranial magnetic resonance imaging of 3,301 elderly people. The Cardiovascular Health Study. Collaborative Researc Group. Neuroepidemiology 2000;19(1):30–42.
[24] Liao D, Cooper L, Cai J, Toole J, Bryan N, Burke G, et al. The prevalence and severity of white matter lesions, their relationship with age, ethnicity, gender, and cardiovascular disease risk factors: the ARIC Study. Neuroepidemiology 1997;16(3):149–62.
[25] Lesser IM, Smith MW, Wohl M, Mena RN, Mehringer CM, Lin KM. Brain imaging, antidepressants, and ethnicity: preliminary observations. Psychopharmacol Bull 1996;32(2): 235–42.
[26] American Psychiatric Association. Diagnostic and statistical manual of mental disorders. 4th edition. Washington, DC: American Psychiatric Press; 1994.
[27] McKhann G, Drachman D, Folstein M, Katzman R, Price D, Stadlan E. Clinical diagnosis of Alzheimer's disease: report of the NINCDS-ADRDA Work Group under the auspices of the Department of Health and Human Services Task Force on Alzheimer's disease. Neurology 1984;34(7):939–44.
[28] Bohnstedt M, Fox PJ, Kohatsu ND. Correlates of Mini-Mental Status Examination scores among elderly demented patients: the influence of race-ethnicity. J Clin Epidemiol 1994; 47(12):1381–7.
[29] Mast BT, Fitzgerald J, Steinberg J, MacNeill SE, Lichtenberg PA. Effective screening for Alzheimer's disease among older African Americans. Clin Neuropsychol 2001;15(2):196–202.
[30] Teresi JA, Albert SM, Holmes D, Mayeux R. Use of latent class analyses for the estimation of prevalence of cognitive impairment, and signs of stroke and Parkinson's disease among African-American elderly of central Harlem: results of the Harlem Aging Project. Neuroepidemiology 1999;18(6):309–21.
[31] Fillenbaum GG, Hughes DC, Heyman A, George LK, Blazer DG. Relationship of health and

demographic characteristics to Mini-Mental State examination score among community residents. Psychol Med 1988;18:719–26.
[32] Escobar JI, Burnam A, Karno M, Forsythe A, Landsverk J, Golding JM. Use of the Mini-Mental State Examination (MMSE) in a community population of mixed ethnicity. Cultural and linguistic artifacts. J Nerv Ment Dis 1986;174(10):607–14.
[33] Welsh KA, Fillenbaum G, Wilkinson W, Heyman A, Mohs RC, Stern Y, et al. Neuropsychological test performance in African-American and white patients with Alzheimer's disease. Neurology 1995;45(12):2207–11.
[34] Kuller LH, Shemanski L, Manolio T, Haan M, Fried L, Bryan N, et al. Relationship between ApoE, MRI findings, and cognitive function in the Cardiovascular Health Study. Stroke 1998; 29(2):388–98.
[35] Salmon DP, Riekkinen PJ, Katzman R, Zhang MY, Jin H, Yu E. Cross-cultural studies of dementia. A comparison of mini-mental state examination performance in Finland and China. Arch Neurol 1989;46(7):769–72.
[36] Overall JE, Levin HS. Correcting for cultural factors in evaluating intellectual deficit on the WAIS. J Clin Psychol 1978;34(4):910–5.
[37] Adams RL, Boake C, Crain C. Bias in a neuropsychological test classification related to education, age, and ethnicity. J Consult Clin Psychol 1982;50(1):143–5.
[38] Jacobs DM, Sano M, Albert S, Schofield P, Dooneief G, Stern Y. Cross-cultural neuropsychological assessment: a comparison of randomly selected, demographically matched cohorts of English- and Spanish-speaking older adults. J Clin Exp Neuropsychol 1997;19(3):331–9.
[39] Kaufman AS, McLean JE, Reynolds CR. Sex, race, residence, region, and education differences on the 11 WAIS-R subtests. J Clin Psychol 1988;44(2):231–48.
[40] Manly JJ, Jacobs DM, Sano M, Bell K, Merchant CA, Small SA, et al. Cognitive test performance among nondemented elderly African Americans and Whites. Neurology 1998;50(5): 1238–45.
[41] Reynolds CR, Chastain RL, Kaufman AS, McLean JE. Demographic characteristics and IQ among adults: Analysis of the WAIS-R standardization sample as a function of the stratification variables. J Sch Psychol 1987;23:323–42.
[42] Roberts RJ, Hamsher KD. Effects of minority status on facial recognition and naming performance. J Clin Psychol 1984;40:539–45.
[43] Ross TP, Lichtenberg PA, Christensen BK. Normative data on the Boston Naming Test for elderly adults in a demographically diverse medical sample. Clin Neuropsychol 1995;9:321–5.
[44] Carlson MC, Brandt J, Carson KA, Kawas CH. Lack of relation between race and cognitive test performance in Alzheimer's disease. Neurology 1998;50(5):1499–501.
[45] Bernard L. Halstead-Reitan neuropsychological test performance of black, Hispanic, and white young adult males from poor academic backgrounds. Arch Clin Neuropsychol 1989;4: 267–74.
[46] Miller EN, Bing EG, Selnes OA, Wesch J, Becker JT. The effects of sociodemographic factors on reaction time and speed of information processing. J Clin Exp Neuropsychol 1993;15:66.
[47] Heverly LL, Isaac W, Hynd GW. Neurodevelopmental and racial differences in tactile-visual (cross-modal) discrimination in normal black and white children. Arch Clin Neuropsychol 1986;1:139–45.
[48] Brown A, Campbell A, Wood D, Hastings A, Lewis-Jack O, Dennis G, et al. Neuropsychological studies of blacks with cerebrovascular disorders: a preliminary investigation. J Natl Med Assoc 1991;83(3):217–24.
[49] Campbell A, Rorie K, Dennis G, Wood D, Combs S, Hearn L, et al. Neuropsychological assessment of African Americans: conceptual and methodological considerations. In: Jones R, editor. Handbook of tests and measurement for black populations, vol. 2. Berkeley, CA: Cobb and Henry; 1996. p. 75–84.
[50] Artiola I, Fortuny L, Heaton RK, Hermosillo D. Neuropsychological comparisons of Spanish-speaking participants from the US-Mexico border region versus Spain. J Int Neuropsychol Soc 1998;4(4):363–79.

[51] Fillenbaum GG, Heyman A, Huber MS, Ganguli M, Unverzagt FW. Performance of elderly African American and white community residents on the CERAD Neuropsychological Battery. J Int Neuropsychol Soc 2001;7(4):502–9.
[52] Ford GR, Haley WE, Thrower SL, West CAC, Harrell LE. Utility of Mini-Mental State Exam scores in predicting functional impairment among white and African American dementia patients. J Gerontol A Biol Sci Med Sci 1996;51(4):185–8.
[53] Marcopulos BA, McLain CA, Giuliano AJ. Cognitive impairment or inadequate norms: a study of healthy, rural, older adults with limited education. Clin Neuropsychol 1997;11:111–31.
[54] Loewenstein DA, Ardila A, Rosselli M, Hayden S. A comparative analysis of functional status among Spanish- and English-speaking patients with dementia. J Gerontol 1992;47(6): P389–94.
[55] Mungas D, Marshall SC, Weldon M, Haan M, Reed BR. Age and education correction of Mini-Mental State Examination for English and Spanish-speaking elderly. Neurology 1996;46(3): 700–6.
[56] Murden RA, McRae TD, Kaner S, Bucknam ME. Mini-Mental State exam scores vary with education in blacks and whites. J Am Geriatr Soc 1991;39(2):149–55.
[57] Ripich DN, Carpenter B, Ziol E. Comparison of African-American and white persons with Alzheimer's disease on language measures. Neurology 1997;48(3):781–3.
[58] Rasmusson DX, Carson KA, Brookmeyer R, Kawas C, Brandt J. Predicting rate of cognitive decline in probable Alzheimer's disease. Brain Cogn 1996;31(2):133–47.
[59] Ford-Booker P, Campbell A, Combs S, Lewis S, Ocampo C, Brown A, et al. The predictive accuracy of neuropsychological tests in a normal population of African Americans. J Clin Exp Neuropsychol 1993;15:64.
[60] Klusman LE, Moulton JM, Hornbostle LK, Picano JJ, Beattie MT. Neuropsychological abnormalities in asymptomatic HIV seropositive military personnel. J Neuropsychiatry Clin Neurosci 1991;3(4):422–8.
[61] Stern Y, Andrews H, Pittman J, Sano M, Tatemichi T, Lantigua R, et al. Diagnosis of dementia in a heterogeneous population. Development of a neuropsychological paradigm-based diagnosis of dementia and quantified correction for the effects of education. Arch Neurol 1992; 49(5):453–60.
[62] Helms JE. Why is there no study of cultural equivalence in standardized cognitive ability testing? Am Psych 1992;47:1083–101.
[63] Ratcliff G, Ganguli M, Chandra V, Sharma S, Belle S, Seaberg E, et al. Effects of literacy and education on measures of word fluency. Brain Lang 1998;61(1):115–22.
[64] Miller SW, Heaton RK, Kirson D, Grant I. Neuropsychological (NP) assessment of African Americans. J Int Neuropsychol Soc 1997;3:49.
[65] Padilla AM. Acculturation: theory, models, and some new findings. Boulder, CO: Westview Press for the American Association for the Advancement of Science; 1980.
[66] Landrine H, Klonoff EA. African American acculturation: deconstructing race and reviving culture. Thousand Oaks, CA: Sage Publications; 1996.
[67] Berry JW. Human ecology and cognitive style. New York: Sage-Halstead; 1976.
[68] Moyerman DR, Forman BD. Acculturation and adjustment - a meta-analytic study. Hisp J Behav Sci 1992;14:163–200.
[69] Negy C, Woods DJ. The importance of acculturation in understanding research with Hispanic-Americans. Hisp J Behav Sci 1992;14:224–47.
[70] Arnold BR, Montgomery GT, Castaneda I, Longoria R. Acculturation and performance of Hispanics on selected Halstead-Reitan neuropsychological tests. Assessment 1994;1:239–48.
[71] Landrine H, Klonoff EA. The African American Acculturation Scale II: cross-validation and short form. J Black Psychol 1995;21:124–52.
[72] Landrine H, Klonoff EA. The African American Acculturation Scale: development, reliability, and validity. J Black Psychol 1994;20:104–27.
[73] Manly JJ, Miller SW, Heaton RK, Byrd D, Reilly J, Velasquez RJ, et al. The effect of African-

American acculturation on neuropsychological test performance in normal and HIV positive individuals. J Int Neuropsychol Soc 1998;4(3):291–302.
[74] Manly JJ, Jacobs DM, Sano M, Bell K, Merchant CA, Small SA, et al. African American acculturation and neuropsychological test performance among nondemented community elders. J Int Neuropsychol Soc 1998;4:77.
[75] Lucas JA. Acculturation and neuropsychological test performance in elderly African Americans. J Int Neuropsychol Soc 1998;4:77.
[76] Kirsch IS, Jungeblut A, Jenkins L, Kolstad A. Adult literacy in America: The National Adult Literacy Survey. National Center for Education Statistics, US Department of Education. Washington, DC: US Government Printing Office; 1993.
[77] Kaufman JS, Cooper RS, McGee DL. Socioeconomic status and health in blacks and whites: the problem of residual confounding and the resilience of race. Epidemiology 1997;8(6): 621–8.
[78] Whitfield KE, Baker-Thomas T. Individual differences in aging minorities. Int J Aging Hum Dev 1999;48(1):73–9.
[79] Loewenstein DA, Arguelles T, Arguelles S, Linn-Fuentes P. Potential cultural bias in the neuropsychological assessment of the older adult. J Clin Exp Neuropsychol 1994;16(4): 623–9.
[80] Margo RA. Disenfranchisement, school finance, and the economics of segregated schools in the United States south, 1980–1910. New York: Garland Publishing; 1985.
[81] Margo RA. Race and schooling in the South, 1880–1950: an economic history. Chicago: University of Chicago Press; 1990.
[82] Smith JP. Race and human capital. Am Econ Rev 1984;4:685–98.
[83] Smith JP, Welch F. Black-White male wage ratios: 1960–1970. Am Econ Rev 1977;67:323–8.
[84] Welch F. Black-White differences in returns to schooling. Am Econ Rev 1973;63:893–907.
[85] Welch F. Measurement of the quality of education. Am Econ Rev 1966;56:379–92.
[86] Weiss BD, Reed R, Kligman EW, Abyad A. Literacy and performance on the Mini-Mental State Examination. J Am Geriatr Soc 1995;43(7):807–10.
[87] Manly JJ, Jacobs DM, Sano M, Bell K, Merchant CA, Small SA, et al. Effect of literacy on neuropsychological test performance in nondemented, education-matched elders. J Int Neuropsychol Soc 1999;5(3):191–202.
[88] Scribner S, Cole M. The psychology of literacy. Cambridge, MA: Harvard University Press; 1981.
[89] Lecours AR, Mehler J, Parente MA, Caldeira A, Cary L, Castro MJ, et al. Illiteracy and brain damage. 1. Aphasia testing in culturally contrasted populations (control subjects). Neuropsychologia 1987;25(1B):231–45.
[90] Reis A, Guerreiro M, Castro-Caldas A. Influence of educational level of non brain-damaged subjects on visual naming capacities. J Clin Exp Neuropsychol 1994;16(6):939–42.
[91] Ardila A, Rosselli M, Rosas P. Neuropsychological assessment in illiterates: visuospatial and memory abilities. Brain Cogn 1989;11(2):147–66.
[92] Rosselli M, Ardila A, Rosas P. Neuropsychological assessment in illiterates. II. Language and praxic abilities. Brain Cogn 1990;12(2):281–96.
[93] Matute E, Leal F, Zaraboso A, Robles A, Cedillo C. Influence of literacy level on stick constructions in non-brain-damaged subjects. J Int Neuropsychol Soc 1997;3:32.
[94] Manly JJ, Jacobs DM, Touradji P, Small SA, Stern Y. Reading level attenuates differences in neuropsychological test performance between African American and white elders. J Int Neuropsychol Soc 2002;8(3):341–8.
[95] Kawas CH, Katzman R. Epidemiology of dementia and Alzheimer's disease. In: Terry RD, Katzman R, Sisodia SS, Bick KL, editors. Alzheimer's disease. Philadelphia: Lippincott Williams & Wilkins; 1999. p. 95–116.
[96] Caramelli P, Poissant A, Gauthier S, Bellavance A, Gauvreau D, Lecours AR, et al. Educational level and neuropsychological heterogeneity in dementia of the Alzheimer type. Alzheimer Dis Assoc Disord 1997;11(1):9–15.

[97] Hill LR, Klauber MR, Salmon DP, Yu ESH, Lui WT, Zhang M, et al. Functional status, education, and the diagnosis of dementia in the Shanghai survey. Neurology 1993;43(1): 138–45.

[98] Zhang M, Katzman R, Salmon D, Jin H, Cai G, Wang Z, et al. The prevalence of dementia and Alzheimer's disease in Shanghai, China: impact of age, gender and education. Ann Neurol 1990;27(4):428–37.

[99] Sulkava R, Wikstrom J, Aromaa A, Raitasalo R, Lahtinen V, Lahtela K, et al. Prevalence of severe dementia in Finland. Neurology 1985;35(7):1025–9.

[100] Dartigues JF, Gagnon M, Michel P, Latenneur L, Commenges D, Barberger-Gateau P, et al. Le programme de recherche paquid sur l'epidemiologie de la demence methodes et resultats initiaux. Rev Neurol (Paris) 1991;147(3):225–30.

[101] Bonaiuto S, Rocca WA, Lippi A, Luciani P, Turtu F, Cavarzeran F, et al. Impact of education and occupation on prevalence of Alzheimer's disease (AD) and multi-infarct dementia (MID) in Appignano, Macerata Province, Italy. Neurology 1990;40(Suppl 1):346.

[102] Prencipe M, Casini AR, Ferretti C, Lattanzio MT, Fiorelli M, Culasso F. Prevalence of dementia in an elderly rural population: effects of age, sex, and education. J Neurol Neurosurg Psychiatry 1996;60(6):628–33.

[103] Korczyn AD, Kahana E, Galper Y. Epidemiology of dementia in Ashkelon, Israel. Neuroepidemiology 1991;10:100.

[104] Bowirrat A, Treves T, Friedland RP, Korczyn AD. Prevalence of Alzheimer's type dementia in an elderly Arab population. Eur J Neurol 2001;8(2):119–23.

[105] Ott A, Breteler MM, van Harskamp F, Claus JJ, van der Cammen TJ, Grobbee DE, et al. Prevalence of Alzheimer's disease and vascular dementia: association with education. The Rotterdam study. Br Med J 1995;310(6985):970–3.

[106] Fratiglioni L, Grut M, Forsell Y, Viitanen M, Grafstrom M, Holmen K, et al. Prevalence of Alzheimer's disease and other dementias in an elderly urban population: relationship with age, sex and education. Neurology 1991;41(12):1886–92.

[107] Gatz M, Svedberg P, Pederson NL, Mortimer JA, Berg S, Johansson B. Education and the risk of Alzheimer's disease: findings from the study of dementia in Swedish twins. J Gerontol B Psychol Sci Soc Sci 2001;56(5):292–300.

[108] Gurland BJ, Wilder D, Cross P, Lantigua R, Teresi JA, Barret V, et al. Relative rates of dementia by multiple case definitions, over two prevalence periods, in three cultural groups. Am J Geriatr Psyhciatr 1995;3:6–20.

[109] Callahan CM, Hall KS, Hui SL, Musick BS, Unverzagt FW, Hendrie HC. Relationship of age, education, and occupation with dementia among a community-based sample of African Americans. Arch Neurol 1996;53(2):134–40.

[110] Mortel KF, Meyer JS, Herod B, Thornby J. Education and occupation as risk factors for dementias of the Alzheimer and ischemic vascular types. Dementia 1995;6(1):55–62.

[111] Stern Y, Gurland B, Tatemichi TK, Tang MX, Wilder D, Mayeux R. Influence of education and occupation on the incidence of Alzheimer's disease. JAMA 1994;271(13):1004–10.

[112] Letenneur L, Commenges D, Dartigues JF, Barberger-Gateau P. Incidence of dementia and Alzheimer's disease in elderly community residents of south-western France. Int J Epidemiol 1994;23(6):1256–61.

[113] Evans DA, Beckett LA, Albert MS, Herbert LE, Scherr PA, Funkenstein HH, et al. Level of education and change in cognitive function in a community population of older persons. Ann Epidemiol 1993;3(1):71–7.

[114] White L, Katzman R, Losonczy K, Salive M, Wallace R, Berkman L, et al. Association of education with incidence of cognitive impairment in three established populations for epidemiologic studies of the elderly. J Clin Epidemiol 1994;47(4):363–74.

[115] Stern Y, Albert S, Tang M-X, Tsai W-Y. Rate of memory decline in AD is related to education and occupation: cognitive reserve? Neurology 1999;53(9):1942–7.

[116] Unverzagt FW, Hui SL, Farlow MR, Hall KS, Hendrie HC. Cognitive decline and education in mild dementia. Neurology 1998;50(1):181–5.

[117] Teri L, McCurry SM, Edland SD, Kukull WA, Larson EB. Cognitive decline in Alzheimer's disease: a longitudinal investigation of risk factors for accelerated decline. J Gerontol A Biol Sci Med Sci 1995;50A(1):M49–55.
[118] Stern Y, Tang MX, Denaro J, Mayeux R. Increased risk of mortality in Alzheimer's disease patients with more advanced educational and occupational attainment. Ann Neurol 1995;37(5): 590–5.
[119] Albert MS, Jones K, Savage CR, Berkman L, Seeman T, Blazer D, et al. Predictors of cognitive change in older persons: MacArthur studies of successful aging. Psychol Aging 1995;10(4): 578–89.
[120] Chodosh J, Reuben DB, Albert MS, Seeman TE. Predicting cognitive impairment in high-functioning community-dwelling older persons: MacArthur studies of successful aging. J Am Geriatr Soc 2002;50(6):1051–60.
[121] Butler SM, Ashford JW, Snowdon DA. Age, education, and changes in the Mini-Mental State Exam scores of older women: findings from the Nun Study. J Am Geriatr Soc 1996; 44(6):675–81.
[122] Farmer ME, Kittner SJ, Rae DS, Bartko JJ, Regier DA. Education and change in cognitive function: the epidemiologic catchment area study. Ann Epidemiol 1995;5(1):1–7.
[123] Christensen H, Korten AE, Jorm AF, Henderson AS, Jacomb PA, Rodgers B, et al. Education and decline in cognitive performance. Compensatory but not protective. Int J Geriatr Psychiatry 1997;12(3):323–30.
[124] Snowdon DA, Ostwald SK, Kane RL. Education, survival and independence in elderly Catholic sisters, 1936–1988. Am J Epidemiol 1989;130(5):999–1012.
[125] Finley GE, Ardila A, Roselli M. Cognitive aging in illiterate Colombian adults: a reversal of the classical aging pattern? Revista Interamericana de Psicologia 1991;25:103–5.
[126] Stern Y. What is cognitive reserve? Theory and research application of the reserve concept. J Int Neuropsychol Soc 2002;8(3):448–60.
[127] Mortimer JA. Do psychosocial risk factors contribute to Alzheimer's disease? In: Henderson AS, Henderson JH, editors. Etiology of dementia of Alzheimer's type. Chichester, UK: John Wiley and Sons; 1988. p. 39–52.
[128] Satz P, Morgenstern H, Miller EN, Selnes OA, McArthur JC, Cohen BA, et al. Low education as a possible risk factor for cognitive abormalities in HIV-1: findings from the Multicenter AIDS Cohort Study (MACS). J Acquir Immune Defic Syndr 1993;6(5):503–11.
[129] Chandra V, Pandav R, Dodge HH, Johnston JM, Belle SH, DeKosky ST, et al. Incidence of Alzheimer's disease in a rural community in India: the Indo-US study. Neurology 2001;57(6): 985–9.
[130] Hendrie HC. Exploration of environmental and genetic risk factors for Alzheimer's disease: the value of cross cultural studies. Curr Dir Psychol Sci 2001;10:98–101.
[131] Hall KS, Gureje O, Gao S, Ogunniyi A, Hui SL, Baiyewu O, et al. Risk factors and Alzheimer's disease: a comparative study of two communities. Aust NZ J Psychiatry 1998;32(5):698–706.
[132] Manly JJ, Touradji P, Tang M-X, Stern Y. Literacy and memory decline among ethnically diverse elders. J Clin Exp Neuropsychol 2003;25(5):680–90.
[133] Steele CM. A threat in the air: how stereotypes shape intellectual identity and performance. Am Psychol 1997;52(6):613–29.
[134] Steele CM, Aronson J. Stereotype threat and the intellectual test performance of African Americans. J Pers Soc Psychol 1995;69(5):797–811.
[135] Spencer SJ, Steele CM, Quinn DM. Stereotype threat and women's math performance. J Exp Soc Psychol 1999;35:4–28.
[136] Aronson J, Lustina MJ, Good C, Keough K, Steele CM, Brown J. When white men can't do math: necessary and sufficient factors in stereotype threat. J Exp Soc Psychol 1999;35:29–46.
[137] Teng EL. Cross-cultural testing and the Cognitive Abilities Screening Instrument. In: Yeo G, Gallagher-Thompson D, editors. Ethnicity and the dementias. Washington, DC: Taylor and Francis; 1996. p. 77–85.
[138] Sano M, Mackell JA, Ponton M, Ferreira P, Wilson J, Pawluczyk S, et al. The Spanish Instru-

ment Protocol: design and implementation of a study to evaluate treatment efficacy instruments for Spanish-speaking patients with Alzheimer's disease. The Alzheimer's Disease Cooperative Study. Alzheimer Dis Assoc Disord 1997;11(Suppl 2):S57–64.
[139] Kempler D, Teng EL, Dick M, Taussig IM, Davis DS. The effects of age, education, and ethnicity on verbal fluency. J Int Neuropsychol Soc 1998;4(6):531–8.
[140] Artiola I, Fortuny L, Mullaney H. Neuropsychology with Spanish speakers: language use and proficiency issues for test development. J Clin Exp Neuropsychol 1997;19(4):615–22.
[141] Brislin RW. Translation and content-analysis of oral and written material. In: Triandis HC, Berry JW, editors. Methodology. Handbook of cross-cultural psychology, vol. 2. Boston: Allyn & Bacon; 1980. p. 389–444.
[142] Brislin RW. Back-translation for cross-cultural research. J Cross Cult Psychol 1970;1:185–216.
[143] van de Vijver F, Hambleton RK. Translating tests: some practical guidelines. Eur Psychol 1996; 1:89–99.
[144] Ponton MO, Satz P, Herrera L, Ortiz F, Urrutia CP, Young R, et al. Normative data stratified by age and education for the Neuropsychological Screening Battery for Hispanics (NeSBHIS): initial report. J Int Neuropsychol Soc 1996;2(2):96–104.
[145] Teng EL, Hasegawa K, Homma A, Imai Y, Larson E, Graves A, et al. The Cognitive Abilities Screening Instrument (CASI): a practical test for cross-cultural epidemiological studies of dementia. Int Psychogeriatr 1994;6(1):45–58.
[146] Mutchler JE, Brallier S. English language proficiency among older Hispanics in the United States. Gerontologist 1999;39(3):310–9.
[147] Yano K, Grove JS, Masaki KH, White LR, Petrovitch H, Chen R, et al. The effects of childhood residence in Japan and testing language on cognitive performance in late life among Japanese American men in Hawaii. J Am Geriatr Soc 2000;48(2):199–204.
[148] Daker-White G, Beattie AM, Gilliard J, Means R. Minority ethnic groups in dementia care: a review of service needs, service provision and models of good practice. Aging Ment Health 2002;6(2):101–8.
[149] LaCalle JJ, Jose J. Forensic psychological evaluations through an interpreter: legal and ethical issues. Am J Forensic Psychol 1987;5(4):29–43.
[150] Ardila A, Rosselli M, Puente AE. Neuropsychological evaluation of the Spanish speaker. New York: Plenum; 1994.
[151] Putsch RW. Cross-cultural communication: the special case for interpreters in health care. JAMA 1985;254(23):3344–8.
[152] Lee LJ, Batal HA, Maselli JH, Kutner JS. Effect of Spanish interpretation method on patient satisfaction in an urban walk-in clinic. J Gen Intern Med 2002;17(8):641–5.
[153] Kamarow E, Lentzner H, Rooks R, Weeks J, Saydah S. Health, United States 1999: health & aging chartbook. Hyattsville, MD: National Center for Health Statistics; 1999.
[154] Lillard L, Rogowski J, Kington R. Long-term determinants of patterns of health insurance coverage in the Medicare population. Gerontologist 1997;37(3):314–23.
[155] Steinman MA, Sands LP, Covinsky KE. Self-restriction of medications due to cost in seniors without prescription coverage. J Gen Intern Med 2001;16(12):793–9.
[156] Wallace SP, Enriquez-Haass V. Availability, accessibility, and acceptability in the evolving health care system for older adults in the United States. Rev Panam Salud Publica 2001; 10(1):18–28.
[157] Cromley EK, Shannon GW. Locating ambulatory medical care facilities for the elderly. Health Serv Res 1986;21(4):499–514.
[158] Shannon GW, Cromley EK, Fink JL. Pharmacy patronage among the elderly: selected racial and geographical patterns. Soc Sci Med 1985;20(1):85–93.
[159] Cluff LE. Problems of the health-impaired elderly: a foundation's experience in geriatrics. J Am Geriatr Soc 1983;31(11):665–72.
[160] Espino DV, Lichtenstein MP, Palmer RR, Hazuda HP. Ethnic differences in Mini-Mental State Examination (MMSE) scores: where you live makes a difference. J Am Geriatr Soc 2001; 49(5):538–48.

[161] LoGiudice D, Hassett A, Cook R, Flicker L, Ames D. Equity of access to a memory clinic in Melbourne? Non-English speaking background attenders are more severely demented and have increased rates of psychiatric disorders. Int J Geriatr Psychiatry 2001;16(3):327–34.
[162] Espino DV, DelAguila D, Parker RW, Lewis R, Mouton CP, Miles TP. Characteristics of Mexican American elders with dementia presenting to a community-based outpatient memory disorders evaluation unit. Ethn Dis 2002;12(4):517–21.
[163] Cooper-Patrick L, Gallo JJ, Gonzales JJ, Vu HT, Powe NR, Nelson C, et al. Race, gender, and partnership in the patient-physician relationship. JAMA 1999;282(6):583–9.
[164] David RA, Rhee M. The impact of language as a barrier to effective health care in an underserved urban Hispanic community. Mt Sinai J Med 1998;65(5–6):393–7.
[165] Waxman MA, Levitt MA. Are diagnostic testing and admission rates higher in non-English-speaking versus English-speaking patients in the emergency department? Ann Emerg Med 2000;36(5):456–61.
[166] Kao AC, Green DC, Zaslavsky AM, Koplan JP, Cleary PD. The relationship between method of physician payment and patient trust. JAMA 1998;280(19):1708–14.
[167] Morrison RS, Zayas LH, Mulvihill M, Baskin SA, Meier DE. Barriers to completion of health care proxies: an examination of ethnic differences. Arch Intern Med 1998;158(22):2493–7.
[168] Hornung CA, Eleazer GP, Strothers III HS, Wieland GD, Eng C, McCann R, et al. Ethnicity and decision-makers in a group of frail older people. J Am Geriatr Soc 1998;46(3):280–6.
[169] Hepburn K, Reed R. Ethical and cultural issues with Native American Elders: end of life decision making. Clin Geriatr Med 1995;11(1):97–112.
[170] Bedolla MA. The principles of medical ethics and their application to the Mexican American elderly patients. Clin Geriatr Med 1995;11(1):131–8.
[171] O'Brien LA, Grisso JA, Maislin G, LaPann K, Krotki KP, Greco PJ, et al. Nursing home residents' preferences for life-sustaining treatments. JAMA 1995;274(22):1775–9.
[172] Eleazer GP, Hornung CA, Egbert CB, Egbert JR, Eng C, Hedgepeth J, et al. The relationship between ethnicity and advance directives in a frail older population. J Am Geriatr Soc 1996;44(8):938–43.
[173] Youn G, Knight BG, Jeong HS, Benton D. Differences in familism values and caregiving outcomes among Korean, Korean American, and white American dementia caregivers. Psychol Aging 1999;14(3):355–64.
[174] Fox K, Hinton WL, Levkoff S. Take up the caregiver's burden: stories of care for urban African American elders with dementia. Cult Med Psychiatry 1999;23(4):501–29.
[175] Dilworth-Anderson P, Gibson BE. The cultural influence of values, norms, meanings, and perceptions in understanding dementia in ethnic minorities. Alzheimer Dis Assoc Disord 2002;16(Suppl 2):S56–63.
[176] Gratton B, Wilson V. Family support systems and the minority elderly: a cautionary analysis. J Gerontol Soc Work 1988;13(1/2):81–93.
[177] Espino DV, Neufeld RR, Mulvihill MK, Libow LS. Hispanic and non-Hispanic elderly on admission to the nursing home: a pilot study. Gerontologist 1988;28(6):821–4.
[178] Olson MC. The heart still beat, but the brain doesn't answer." Perception and experience of old-age dementia in the Milwaukee Hmong community. Theor Med Bioeth 1999;20(1):85–95.
[179] Weintraub D, Raskin A, Ruskin PE, Gruber-Baldini AL, Zimmerman SI, Hebel JR, et al. Racial differences in the prevalence of dementia among patients admitted to nursing homes. Psychiatr Serv 2000;51(10):1259–64.
[180] Wallace SP, Levy-Storms L, Kington RS, Andersen RM. The persistence of race and ethnicity in the use of long-term care. J Gerontol B Psychol Sci Soc Sci 1998;53(2):S104–12.
[181] Lakdawalla D, Goldman DP, Bhattacharya J, Hurd MD, Joyce GF, Panis CW. Forecasting the nursing home population. Med Care 2003;41(1):8–20.
[182] Huber R, Borders K, Netting FE, Nelson HW. Data from long-term care ombudsman programs in six states: the implications of collecting resident demographics. Gerontologist 2001;41(1):61–8.

[183] Bernabei R, Gambassi G, Lapane K, Landi F, Gatsonis C, Dunlop R, et al. Management of pain in elderly patients with cancer. SAGE Study Group. Systematic assessment of geriatric drug use via epidemiology. JAMA 1998;279(23):1877–82.

[184] Li PL, Logan S, Yee L, Ng S. Barriers to meeting the mental health needs of the Chinese community. J Public Health Med 1999;21(1):74–80.

[185] Krakauer EL, Crenner C, Fox K. Barriers to optimum end-of-life care for minority patients. J Am Geriatr Soc 2002;50(1):182–90.

[186] Carrese JA, Rhodes LA. Western bioethics on the Navajo reservation. JAMA 1995;274(10): 826–9.

[187] Blackhall LJ, Frank G, Murphy ST, Michel V, Palmer JM, Azen SP. Ethnicity and attitudes towards life sustaining technology. Soc Sci Med 1999;48(12):1779–89.

[188] Akabayashi A, Fetters MD, Elwyn TS. Family consent, communication, and advance directives for cancer disclosure: a Japanese case and discussion. J Med Ethics 1999;25(4):296–301.

[189] Mebane EW, Oman RF, Kroonen LT, Goldstein MK. The influence of physician race, age, and gender on physician attitudes toward advance care directives and preferences for end-of-life decision-making. J Am Geriatr Soc 1999;47(5):579–91.

[190] Crawley LM, Marshall PA, Lo B, Koenig BA. The End-of-Life Care Consensus Panel. Strategies for culturally effective end-of-life care. Ann Intern Med 2002;136(9):673–9.

ELSEVIER
SAUNDERS

Clin Geriatr Med 20 (2004) 121–139

CLINICS IN
GERIATRIC
MEDICINE

Interdisciplinary approaches to Alzheimer's disease management

Elizabeth A. Crooks, RN, MSN, CCRN, CS[a],
David S. Geldmacher, MD[b,*]

[a]*Frances Payne Bolton School of Nursing, Case Western Reserve University, 10900 Euclid Avenue, Cleveland, OH 44106, USA*
[b]*Department of Neurology, University of Virginia Health System, P.O. Box 800394, Charlottesville, VA 22908, USA*

The needs of the patient with dementia are extensive, and pharmacologic management of the illness is limited. The clinical syndrome of Alzheimer's disease (AD) is treatable, but its management is complex and extends beyond the traditional bounds of medical practice. Whereas medicine has historically focused on effects of disease on the patient, dementia treatment requires a broader focus on the effect of the symptoms on the patient and those who provide care for the patient. This requires attention to the quality of the lives of the affected people (ie, both the patient and the caregivers) to a greater extent than most other disease states. Many of the most effective interventions are nonpharmacologic and may be provided by professionals from multiple disciplines. Families who cope with dementing illness often seek services from several health care providers, social service agencies, and professionals from outside of health care such as lawyers and financial planners. Often the primary care physician must direct the family to obtain these services. Linking the patient to skills and resources available in the community can dramatically reduce the care burden to the family and the doctor.

This review provides the clinician with the necessary information to effectively use an interdisciplinary approach to care for the patient with dementia. It uses a case-based approach to focus attention on the patient and caregiver experience when living with AD. Strategies to identify problems amenable to interdisciplinary intervention are discussed, and team member responsibilities are described. Referral suggestions are made for common problems associated with dementing illness.

* Corresponding author.
E-mail address: dsg8n@virginia.edu (D.S. Geldmacher).

doi:10.1016/j.cger.2003.11.004

Challenges to medical practice

Management of AD presents unique challenges to the practicing clinician. Although pharmacologic intervention such as cholinesterase inhibitors or NMDA receptor antagonist approaches may delay the loss of cognitive function and decrease difficult behavioral symptoms, successful management of AD and other progressive dementias hinges on a team approach that moves beyond the boundaries of medical practice. This approach relies less on standard pharmacologically based medical practice and more on the integration of therapies from a wide range of health care providers and community professionals. To implement this approach effectively, the physician must understand the caregiving experience and how the caregiver burden influences patient care. The clinician must be informed about the resources available to meet the medical, social, economic, and emotional needs of the patient within the context of their family and community. Using the multidisciplinary team approach to patient care can be complex, but it benefits both the patient and the clinician. It allows the physician to focus on issues that are most likely to respond to medical intervention, while it anticipates and manages patient problems that are likely to trigger frequent calls for assistance.

The caregiver experience

Mr. K is an 82-year-old man who was diagnosed with AD approximately 2 years ago. He is being managed with a cholinesterase inhibitor and presents to his primary care physician for a follow-up evaluation. He now lives with his 53-year-old son and daughter-in-law. The daughter-in-law accompanies him to see the physician. Mr. K denies medical complaints and states that he is doing well at home. He has a pleasant affect, appears well nourished and well groomed, and cooperates with the examination. His daughter-in-law relates that although Mr. K does not perceive that he is doing poorly, over the last 2 months he has become intermittently incontinent of urine. Recently he had a single episode of bowel incontinence and was unable to clean himself properly. She also relates that her father-in-law seems to be more easily distracted from other activities of daily living (ADLs) such as grooming and eating and now requires assistance in the completion of these tasks. One week before this visit the patient's son found Mr. K agitated and pounding on the garage door. He was unable to operate the automated door-opener and apparently had forgotten he could use the doorway directly back to the living quarters. Fearful for Mr. K's safety, she has reluctantly agreed to take a leave of absence from her job so that Mr. K is not left unsupervised at home.

The patient–caregiver relationship

Mr. K's daughter-in-law faces several problems typical to caregivers. As Mr. K's function declines, the burden of his care increases and now impacts heavily on his daughter-in-law's personal and professional life. This burden includes economic considerations as the family's income declines due to a change in the daughter-in-law's employment. Whereas it is prudent to rule out the contribution of a medical condition to Mr. K's functional decline, it is also imperative to address how the family plans to manage Mr. K's continued loss of independence as the disease progresses.

Medical care commonly focuses on diagnosis and management of an impaired individual. When a team approach is implemented, the focus of care expands to include the patient's caregiver. For the vast majority of patients with AD, the caregiver is someone within the family, 73% of the time a woman who provides care informally and without compensation [1,2]. The patient's spouse often assumes the role of caregiver, although it is common, as in the case of Mr. K, for the caregiver to be the patient's adult daughter or daughter-in-law. These family members have been called the "hidden victims" of AD because they must handle the physical, social, and emotional consequences of the disease [3]. Most of the time, the caregiver strives to preserve or enhance the patient's quality of life within their family and community. The interdisciplinary team's goal is to optimize the patient's ability to function within his or her family, as well as to support the caregiver and other family members in their efforts to maintain a safe and satisfying environment.

Gender differences appear to have a significant impact on the caregiver experience, so it is important to note that the majority of caregivers are women. In American culture, men and women are socialized very differently to caregiving roles. Traditionally, women are expected to assume caregiving duties with minimal assistance from male family members [4]. Because many caregivers are invested in the cultural tradition that a woman's role is concentrated in the home, it is easy to understand how obtaining support from outside sources to help balance work and family responsibilities may be overlooked [5]. These women perform the stressful duties of custodial and emotional patient care and frequently view their caregiving role as both an obligation and a labor of love. They sacrifice their own needs while feelings of anger, pain, and resentment are suppressed. Furthermore, they may feel intense guilt if they acknowledge these emotions. Men, on the other hand, are more likely to approach the job of caregiving through delegation of duties and access to outside services for both household and patient management. They tend to have a task-oriented approach that includes a plan that allows a balance of work, rest, and leisure [4].

All caregivers, regardless of gender and approach to patient management, experience emotional and physical strain. Cardiovascular problems such as hypertension and myocardial infarction have been reported along with gastric ulcers and immune compromise [6]. Clinical depression has been found to develop in about half of the primary caregivers and, not surprisingly, it worsens as the patient's disease progresses [7]. Other common caregiver problems include disrupted sleep, fatigue, and appetite and weight changes. As the patient's ability to function declines, the caregivers find themselves taking on an even larger role in meeting the patient's physical and emotional needs. When behavioral symptoms related to AD emerge, such as agitation, wandering, day/night reversal, and paranoid ideation, meeting the patient's physical needs becomes more difficult. Caregivers find their personal resources and ability to cope become exhausted and they are less able to deal with their emotional responses to caregiving. These responses include feelings of anger, helplessness, and social isolation [8]. Assumption of caregiving also has the potential to change family dynamics and requires family members to take on roles for which they may be ill prepared. As family dynamics change, longstanding conflicts may be exacerbated and new conflicts may arise. The impact on patient management is obvious. As caregivers reach their limit to solve problems unassisted, they seek help from the primary care provider. To assist the patient and their family adequately, it is necessary to assess the caregiver's social, emotional, and physical resources. One tool for assessing caregiver strain, the Margaret Blenkner Research Center Caregiver Strain Instrument, is available on line at http://www.nccconline.org/pdf/CCN-AD_tools6-03.pdf.

Interdisciplinary team construction, leadership, and member contributions

Miss Y is a 76-year-old retired church secretary who was diagnosed with AD three years ago. Miss Y refuses to take medications because she considers them not to be "part of God's plan." She recently sold her home on the advice of her attorney, placed her assets in a living trust, and has moved in with her niece's family. Miss Y's niece reports that her aunt has frequent periods of agitation and will often accuse her of trying to steal her money. She also is having difficulty adapting to living in her niece's house, which she finds loud and "unmannerly." Miss Y regularly demands to be taken home. She becomes distraught when she is reminded that she now lives with her niece. Her niece is worried that the stress of having her aunt living in her house will negatively impact on her marriage and children. Miss Y's niece regularly attends a support group sponsored by The Alzheimer's Association, which she reports as helpful. She is concerned that her family's quality of life is progressively declining as a result of her aunt's constant dissatisfaction and unpredictable behavior. She is considering recommending that her Aunt move to a faith-based retirement community that is able to provide her with assisted living.

Multidisciplinary versus interdisciplinary approaches

The best approach to care of the AD patient population includes support from multiple sources. These sources may be integrated, parallel, or both. It is ideal for patients and their families to seek a blend of multidisciplinary and interdisciplinary care. These services may come from various health care providers, social service agencies, and professionals from outside of health care.

Multidisciplinary care differs from interdisciplinary care by the amount of interaction that occurs among providers. Multidisciplinary care refers to the delivery of parallel services without direct interaction between providers. A person who sees a doctor, attends a support group, and obtains legal advice from an attorney with little or no interaction among these providers receives multidisciplinary care. Interdisciplinary care involves the use of a team where providers collaborate to identify and meet patient needs. Ideally this team is composed of a physician, nurse, social worker, and other allied health specialists as needed. Because interdisciplinary team members have areas of practice that overlap, team leadership is enhanced when the members understand each other's contributions and expertise.

Team structure

Interdisciplinary teams can be structured either formally or informally. A team with informal structure varies membership and leadership based on individual patient need, and the members' responsibilities may overlap. Team construction is dictated by time, commitment from the organization or practice group, as well as financial and human resources. Regardless of structure, successful teams are characterized by a shared commitment to quality care and an appreciation for the contributions of each member [9].

Conflict is inherent to any team effort, so team coordination requires not only time but also strong organizational and communication skills. Team leadership may fall to any team member; however, use of a registered nurse or social worker as the team leader frees the physician to focus on medical management. Interdisciplinary case management services are available in many communities. These services can be accessed through hospital-based social services departments, home health care agencies, charitable organizations, or proprietary case management companies. Local chapters of the Alzheimer's Association are also a good resource for suggestions and help with coordination of dementia-related services.

Team members

The physician

The physician's primary responsibility is diagnosis of the dementing illness using validated criteria and practice guidelines. After diagnosis, the physician determines prognosis and prescribes medicines to treat the disease and underlying symptoms. When the demented individual does not meet diagnostic criteria or if diagnostic certainty is low, referral to a subspecialist who has expertise in dementia, behavioral neurology, or neuropsychiatry may be useful to refine the diagnostic certainty and help develop a plan of care. As an alternative to physician care, a neuropsychologist may be consulted. These clinicians interpret quantitative cognitive performance data and report it to the referring physician. Many also provide ongoing counseling and support to the patient and family. Medical schools and academic facilities are a good resource for finding appropriate subspecialists.

The physician is also frequently responsible for providing the family and patient with appropriate referrals for management of problems that cannot be addressed by pharmacologic therapies. The National Chronic Care Consortium (NCCC) in cooperation with the Alzheimer's Association has identified guidelines for the interdisciplinary management of patients suffering from dementia. These guidelines take into account disease progression and describe strategies to be used at the time of diagnosis, during long-term management, and at end of life [2]. They are available for download at http://www.nccconline.org/pdf/CCN-AD_tools6-03.pdf.

The nurse

The nurse's role in caring for the demented person and their caregivers varies based on the nurse's licensure and scope of practice. The registered nurse (RN) is primarily responsible for the assessment and management of the patient and caregivers' response to the dementing illness. This includes monitoring symptoms and patient response to medication, meeting the education needs of the patient and their caregivers, and assisting them in preparing for disease progression. Professional nursing practice is based on a conceptual framework that focuses care toward the patient within the broader context of their family and community. This philosophic orientation fits well with the management of the patient with dementia. In many institutions the RN acts as a case manager or interdisciplinary team leader and initiates referrals to address medical, emotional, and social problems associated with the illness.

Along with social workers, registered nurses are skilled at managing the patient and caregivers' psychosocial needs. Registered nurses are ideally qualified to implement the NCCC and the Alzheimer's Association guidelines for meeting the functional and psychosocial needs of the patient with dementia. In practice settings that do not use RNs, access to an RN for case management can be done with a referral to a hospital-based home care program or to an independent home health agency such as Visiting Nurses.

Nurse practitioners (NPs) and clinical nurse specialists (CNSs) are RNs with a Master's degree, clinical doctorate, or PhD, whose scope of practice includes diagnosis of disease and prescription of medications. These advanced practice nurses also have formal education in the research process and may be involved in clinical trials and other methods of scientific inquiry. Advanced practice nurses may be found in solo private practice or in group practices that include physician partners. The scope of practice for these nurses is defined by each state's board of nursing and varies among states. NPs and CNSs provide a cost-effective approach to management of patients with chronic illness.

A licensed practical nurse (LPN) is trained to provide custodial care, carry out treatments, and administer oral and intravenous medications. These nurses have completed a postsecondary training program and are licensed by the state's board of nursing. The LPN may collect patient data such as physical presentation and vital signs but is not qualified to evaluate the data. Because of this inability to provide an evaluative assessment, the LPN must work under the direct supervision of a physician or RN. The LPN is, however, a good choice for providing in-home custodial care for patients with skilled nursing needs.

Nursing care technicians or assistants are unlicensed personnel who focus on custodial care. Their responsibilities vary based on their work setting. Nursing care technicians in long-term care settings not only provide custodial care but may also collect patient data such as vital signs and glucometer readings. In some facilities they may perform simple procedures such as uncomplicated dressing changes. In acute care settings they may perform more complex procedures such as urinary catheterization and venipuncture. In the home care setting these assistants focus on direct patient care such as feeding and bathing and may assume responsibility for light housekeeping and meal preparation.

The social worker

Social workers base their practice on the philosophy that the individual is part of a larger system, and they are prepared to assist the patient and family in acquiring the resources needed to cope with the burden of chronic illness [10]. Because the person with a dementing illness and their caregivers will eventually require access to social services such as respite care, financial services, counseling, or crisis management, a referral to a social worker should occur at the time of diagnosis.

As AD progresses, the patient and family will require increasing levels of support. The social worker is able to assist the patient and family to anticipate future needs, identify community agencies available to meet the patient's complex medical, nursing, and social needs, and guide them through the bureaucracy of health care reimbursement.

AD is chronic, debilitating, and socially isolating. The emotional toll on the family is enormous, and the patient's progressive dependence alters family dynamics. As family dynamics change, unresolved emotional issues exacerbate and new conflicts arise. Hostility may emerge and the risk for elder abuse increases [11,12]. Although all health care professionals must be sensitive to the signs of elder abuse, the social worker's focus on family relationships and dynamics put them in a good position to detect it. Social workers are also skilled in counseling people who find themselves facing role changes, relationship conflict, or are in crisis. In addition, social workers are able to recognize overt psychopathology and can collaborate with physicians and mental health agencies to get psychiatric care for patients or caregivers. As the dementing illness moves into advanced stages, social workers may collaborate with clergy and the patients' attorney to assist the family with long-term placement and end-of-life decisions [10].

The physical therapist

Progressive dementing illnesses frequently result in immobility, decreased physical conditioning, loss of muscle strength and tone, and poor coordination. Impaired ambulation is common and increases the risk for patient falls and injury.

Physical therapy (PT) helps to optimize the patient's physical condition and maintain safe ambulation as long as possible. This ability to maintain the patient's safety is a key factor in keeping the patient at home rather than placement in a long-term care facility.

An exercise and activity plan is developed by the physical therapist and shared with the patient and caregiver. The ability of the patient to comply with the plan often rests with the caregiver, and therefore caregiver education is essential. The physical therapist will also evaluate the need for assistive devices and instruct the patient and caregiver in their use.

PT can occur in the home or in a clinic setting. Where the PT occurs is less important than the patient's ability to learn or comply with the activity plan. In moderate to advanced stages of illness, the benefit of PT may be limited because the patient's ability to follow direction is impaired [13]. Dementing illnesses also alter how a patient interprets changes in the environment. The patient's ability to tolerate environmental changes and their response to social interaction with unfamiliar people should be considered when choosing in-home versus clinic settings.

The occupational therapist

Another important factor in maintaining the patient at home is their ability to manage ADLs. Occupational therapy (OT) plays an important role in aiding the patient and caregiver to adapt to the patient's diminishing ability to manage daily living. Use of assistive devices for toileting, eating, dressing, and home management can be recommended and demonstrated by an OT. As patient independence is enhanced, caregiver burden is eased.

The patient's independence is also influenced by the ability to drive. Unfortunately, dementing illnesses impair driving ability, and even in the face of common sense, many people resist losing this privilege. Formal evaluation of driving skills by an OT may aid in defusing an issue that is emotionally charged for most patients and their families. A driving evaluation clinic provides an unbiased assessment of the patient's abilities. Many rehabilitation hospitals offer formal driving evaluation programs that give a more sophisticated assessment of the patient's driving ability than state motor vehicle departments or commercial driving schools.

The nutritionist

Cognitive impairment related to dementia places the patient at risk for malnutrition and dehydration. In later stages of AD, the patient experiences sensory-motor impairment with ensuing loss of the ability to swallow or eat independently. Weight loss, then, becomes a serious problem as the disease progresses [14]. Comorbid conditions common to the elderly such as diabetes or heart failure also make dietary management difficult. Dietary intake, however, goes beyond medical concern and becomes an important quality of life issue.

Relaxation of restrictive dietary plans should be considered when addressing the patient's quality of life. Unpalatable low sodium or low fat diets may be eliminated in favor of improved caloric intake. This approach is acceptable because AD may impair taste perception and progressive weight loss characterizes the disease. Finally, AD, rather than cardiovascular morbidity, is the primary determinant of life expectancy in this patient population.

A registered dietician is able to assess a patient's nutritional needs and create a plan with the family to ensure that the patient receives adequate calories. They also are able to explore the role food has in the family's life and develop a strategy that incorporates food preferences and family ritual. Food has emotional and social meaning beyond nutrition. A successful approach to patient nutrition maintains the patient's ideal body weight and nutritional well-being without compromising quality of life. When the patient's illness progresses to the point that the patient becomes increasingly malnourished, the registered dietician can be a valuable resource to family decision-making about nutritional support at end of life.

The clergy member

Humans are spiritual beings. The majority of elderly persons (75%) are members of a religious organization although they may not regularly attend formal services or meetings [15]. Organized religion provides a framework for understanding the meaning of existence; however, it is not a requirement for people to feel spiritually fulfilled. The diagnosis of a serious illness, particularly one that is not curable and will result in disability and death, may predispose the patient, caregiver, and other family members to spiritual distress.

Spiritual distress manifests itself several ways. Commonly, people question the meaning of life, death, suffering, and the credibility of their belief system [16]. Feelings of anger, resentment, and fear may also be experienced. Spiritual distress may result in the person's withdrawal from the usual practice of religious rituals. Withdrawal from religious practice may also occur involuntarily due to the social isolation inherent to progressive dementia.

The spiritual resources available to the patient become increasingly important as the family works through end of life issues. Consultation with clergy is helpful when patients and their caregivers face life-prolonging options in the face of disease advancement. Families must make decisions regarding care and the treatment of potentially life-threatening illnesses as they arise. They not only witness but participate in the patient's dying [6]. Clergy and lay ministers help the family members address these ethical issues within the context of their faith and culture. They also are able to marshal resources within the religious community to support the patient and caregiver.

Clergy are an excellent resource for grief management and bereavement care. Patients with dementia and their families face continuous loss throughout the disease process. They must cope with the loss of cognitive and physical function as well as the loss of relationships and social standing. They must deal with the grief of current losses while anticipating greater losses in the future.

Clergy aid the family and patient to make sense of this experience, assign it meaning, and proceed with grief.

Ideally, the patient and family should be referred for spiritual guidance to the spiritual leader of their religious community with whom they already have a relationship. When this isn't feasible, the patient and caregiver should be informed of options for pastoral care available from the chaplain or department of pastoral care at their local hospital, the local chapter of the National Council of Churches, or from their local chapter of the Alzheimer's Association.

The lawyer

Safeguarding the social and economic well-being of the patient and family is an important interdisciplinary concern. The costs of care and the loss of mental capacity from AD have serious legal implications for both patients and their families. Consultation with an attorney that specializes in elder or family law is strongly advised at diagnosis. The attorney makes an important contribution to the patient's care by guiding plans for disability. Legal services are focused on safeguarding the patient's and family's assets, protection from abuse and exploitation, and preserving the patient's rights.

As dementia progresses, the patient's capacity diminishes. Capacity is the ability to understand the nature and consequences of one's actions. It is a fundamental tenet in contract formation, will execution, and the commission of criminal acts. A person with AD may or may not be incapacitated. Over time, however, the person's ability to understand and retain new information, problem solve, behave appropriately, and communicate becomes impaired. At some point the patient with AD will lose the ability to make competent decisions. Although it is painful for the family and patient to anticipate the loss of self-determination, it is very important that discussions regarding capacity begin while the patient still has the ability to identify the person they would like to act as guardian. This is an emotion-laden decision that should be made early in the disease course. Creating a mechanism that provides for substitute decision-making is of primary concern for the patient with AD [17]. This can be done by establishing a guardianship, conservatorship, power of attorney, or trust [18]. Another means of safeguarding the patient's wishes is the establishment of advance directives. Designing a legal plan can be difficult, however, because the attorney must take into account the patient's capacity.

Before the initiation of a legal action, the attorney must determine if the patient has sufficient capacity to retain him or her and whether that judgment is enough to meet the goals of representation [17]. The person must have the ability to articulate the reasons behind decisions and understand the consequences of those decisions. Consultation with the patient's physician is essential when the attorney is uncertain of a patient's capacity.

Although the most urgent legal considerations for the patient with AD involve providing a means to safeguard patients' rights and ensure their voice in directing their own care, an attorney is also valuable in protecting the patient's assets. Issues such as estate planning, asset inventory, and plans for asset transfer after death require examination. Existing legal claims should be reviewed, and the patient and family should be counseled as to the ability of the patient to enter into future contracts. Finally, an attorney can coordinate background investigations of candidates for employment within the home.

Evaluating caregiver burden

Caregivers experience complex emotions that may make it difficult for them to admit to problems during an office interview. This makes determining which services the patient and family could benefit from a challenge. A statement that allows the caregiver the freedom to express their frustrations with patient care should be made with each office visit. This giving of "permission" to speak freely may allow them to be candid about how they are dealing with the stressors at home.

Contrary to what many would expect, a linear relationship between caregiver burden and patient impairment has not been supported in the literature [19]. Caregiver burden is multifactorial and linked to variables such as availability of social support and financial resources, coping abilities, and feelings of self-efficacy [20]. Because it is difficult to predict which caregivers require assistance, it is prudent to use a standardized assessment tool to uncover and focus discussion on current or anticipated problems.

The emotional and physical costs of caregiving are enormous. It is important, then, to create a patient care plan that conserves caregiver resources, anticipates future needs, recognizes caregiver limitations, and sets boundaries for caregiver self-sacrifice. To accomplish this, the health care provider must have a good understanding of common problems that the patient and caregiver face and the means used to uncover them.

Functional assessment

Mrs. A is a moderately obese 73-year-old woman with a history of hypertension, type II diabetes, and osteoporosis. She has cognitive and functional impairments consistent with early stage AD. Her blood pressure has been previously well maintained on a combined β-blocker/diuretic; her serum glucose levels are stable with an oral hypoglycemic agent. Alendronate was begun ~ 1 year ago to maintain bone density. On the advice of a neurologist, Mrs. A has also been taking a cholinesterase inhibitor and vitamin E for her AD. She presents to the primary care physician accompanied by her son who is concerned that his mother's memory has worsened. As a result he has been giving her gingko biloba. He states that his mother is impaired in her ability to cook and clean. He is finding empty soup cans in the kitchen but little evidence of other shopping or cooking. He is concerned about the impact of "all that sodium." Several times, he has found rotting produce in the refrigerator crisper drawer, which is out of character for his mother. He is now managing her finances after finding her checking account $1500 overdrawn from multiple donations to local fire companies and police organizations. He also is concerned that Mrs. A may not be remembering to take her medications as prescribed. Mrs. A, on the other hand, is unconcerned about her ability to maintain her household. While she admits to being forgetful, she states that she is able to cook, clean, and run errands without problems.

AD is characterized by the patient's lack of insight regarding self-care deficits. As dementia progresses, patients become less able to function within their family and community and at the same time are unaware of the extent of their disability. It is important that the patient is not the sole informant during office visits. Family and caregiver impressions of how the patient is managing are crucial to the development of a team-centered plan.

Assessment of patient problems is focused in two different areas. The first is evaluation of actual physical, emotional, and social difficulties. These are problems that the patient or family is coping with now. The second area is evaluation of problems that have the potential to arise as the illness advances. This can be difficult because there is no way to predict how and when a person will lose function. It is certain, however, that they will. Mrs. A's case demonstrates someone who has difficulties with bill payment. It is also likely that she has lost her ability to use her medicines safely, especially something with a relatively complicated regimen like alendronate. Because she lives alone, it is reasonable to assume that Mrs. A may have additional problems that no one has noticed. Consideration of potential problems along with actual problems provides a prospective rather than reactive framework for patient care. Anticipation of problems also allows for early referral and more effective patient management. Box 1 suggests some areas to assess for potential problems.

Screening for problems in daily function

The history and physical customarily focus on the patient's physical presentation leaving emotional and social issues unexamined. A mechanism for diagnosing nonphysiologic problems that are amendable to a team approach is required. One way to accomplish this is through the use of standardized screening tools coupled with a caregiver/family interview. The Agency for Health Care Policy and Research (AHCPR) Practice Guideline for the early identification of dementia [21] recommends that initial assessment of functional impairment be done using the Functional Activities Questionnaire (FAQ) [1]. The FAQ is available on the NCCC web site (http://www.nccconline.org/pdf/CCN-AD_tools6-03.pdf). An FAQ score of 9 or more, showing dependency in three or more activities, indicates functional impairment that requires further evaluation. Screening for problems using the FAQ does not require a physician. A nurse, social worker, or other medical staff may administer it, and the findings are useful for guiding the caregiver interview. This approach saves physician time and

Box 1. Questions to assess patient/caregiver psychosocial needs and resources

Financial needs and resources

- Have your insurance policies been reviewed recently?
- Do you have a mechanism for bill payment and money management?
- Is there someone who is able to help you with business decisions?
- Does this person know what your financial plan is and how to access help for you when you need it?
- Do you expect to hire in-home assistance when you can no longer manage housekeeping or personal tasks for yourself?

Social needs and resources

- How do you spend your leisure time?
- Are you able to stay in touch with family and friends?
- Who do you can count on for help when you need it?
- Has AD changed your ability to socialize with the people you consider important?

Legal needs and resources

- Do you have an attorney?
- Is your estate planning complete?
- Do you have any legal claims pending?
- Do you have an advance directive (living will) that identifies a health care proxy?
- Have you recently entered into a contract that has not been reviewed by an attorney?
- Is your will up-to-date?

Spiritual needs and resources

- Are you a member of a formal religious organization?
- Are you able to maintain your usual religious activities?
- Do you find your religious group supportive?
- Do you have a spiritual leader?
- Are you comfortable contacting your spiritual leader for assistance in managing the demands of caregiving or coping with the losses from AD?

keeps discussions focused so that patient and caregiver problems can be addressed more effectively. Although the FAQ is not diagnostic of AD, it provides clues regarding the types of services the patient or caregiver may need. In Mrs. A's case, her difficulties in managing financial affairs may indicate a need for a legal referral. If problems with meal planning and preparation are confirmed, an occupational therapist, nutritionist, or custodial nursing referral may be considered.

The Index of ADL [22] allows the clinician to assess the patient's ability to complete complex tasks. It is also available at http://www.nccconline.org/pdf/CCN-AD_tools6-03.pdf. The instrument is structured to provide specific information regarding the patient's ability to manage self-care activities such as toileting, grooming, eating, and ambulation and identifies the level of assistance the caregiver lends. This provides not only useful information regarding patient function but also caregiver burden. Whereas other scales may also provide useful additional information, the economy of words used in the Index of ADL may be quite useful when working with individuals who have difficulty reading.

Standardized assessment tools such as the FAQ and Index of ADL are inexpensive, easy to administer by a nonphysician staff member, and do a good job of providing information about how the patient and caregiver are coping with the challenges of living with dementia. They are limited, however, in identifying potential problems because they only measure current function. In essence, they provide a snapshot of the present. They do not take into account what the patient and family will face in the future. They also do not provide information regarding the patient's psychosocial well-being. It is important, then, to supplement the FAQ and Index of ADLs with future-oriented questions to help the patient and caregiver consider what their present resources are and what they may be in the future.

Analyzing the data

It is important to confirm and clarify responses given on assessment tools both during the patient/caregiver interview and by directly observing the patient. A clear understanding of what the patients and their families think and feel enhances the clinician's ability to mobilize the interdisciplinary team and address problems as soon as they are identified. Finally, it is important to remember that the patient and their family members are dealing with more than the loss of physical and cognitive ability. It is important to explore the meaning of these losses to the individual and their emotional reaction to them [11].

Integration of community resources into the care plan

Mr. G is a 69-year-old man with a 4-year history of AD. He has a history of hypertension and chronic renal failure. He has been managed for the last 2 years on a cholinesterase inhibitor. He presents to his primary physician accompanied by his wife and adult son. The family relates that Mr. G seems apathetic and depressed. He no longer tends to his rose garden and his appetite is poor. Mr. G usually sleeps on and off through the day while sitting in front of the television. At night he becomes irritable and will stay awake until the early morning hours. Mrs. G appears exhausted and states that she rarely gets more than 3 or 4 hours of sleep at night. Mr. G's son has offered to have his father stay at his home while his mother rests and visits her out of town sister. Mrs. G refuses and states that her husband would not be happy without her. She also claims that her husband does not get along with their son's wife.

Meeting patient and caregiver information needs

It is not uncommon for patients or their families to present to their health care provider armed with information gleaned from popular magazines, television, or the Internet. Unfortunately, the accuracy and quality of this information varies, and it takes time to help the patient and family make sense of information that comes from these sources. A library of written materials from valid sources can help to reinforce the information provided during brief patient/caregiver visits and introduce them to available community resources. Written materials also allow the family to review the information at their leisure and refer to it in the future. Many chapters of the Alzheimer's Association maintain this sort of information.

Using community resources

Community resources can be invaluable in meeting patient and caregiver needs; however, availability of programs and services will vary by region. Formal resources such as local chapters of the Alzheimer's Association can be found in most urban and many rural areas. The American Association of Retired Persons (AARP) has a network of local chapters with experienced volunteers who can assist patients and caregivers to access services specifically for people coping with AD and related disorders. Other helpful programs include state or local offices of aging. Community offices of aging use federal, state, local, and private funds to administer services for older adults and their caregivers. Because these services vary by community, patients/caregivers should contact their local office of aging for a list of services designed for people with dementing illness.

Informal sources of support are available in most communities. These include church groups, concerned neighbors, and extended family members. The increased availability of Internet access also allows families to obtain information and create support networks informally.

The Alzheimer's Association

The Alzheimer's Association is a national organization whose mission is to support patients with AD and their caregivers. It acts as a clearinghouse for information and sponsors programs for health care providers. Local chapters offer programs and publications to educate patients and caregivers about medical issues, and they advocate for people with dementing illnesses. Structured support groups and referral to other community resources are also available through local chapters.

Local chapters frequently provide educational program to inform and support early- to middle-stage caregivers. This usually includes a medical overview, approaches to manage behavioral issues, and suggestions for meeting custodial care needs. This type of educational support helps the family anticipate and plan for the long-term consequences of the disease and may reduce the demands for the physician to provide similar information in medical office visits.

The Safe Return program is a nationwide service sponsored by the Alzheimer's Association to help police and private citizens identify, locate, and return people with dementia. Caregivers of patients at risk for wandering should register their loved ones with Safe Return. Safe Return provides an identification item (wallet card, jewelry, or clothing label) for the registered person. This item provides a national 800 number that is accessible to operators 24 hours a day, 7 days a week. When a person who is registered in the program becomes lost, his or her family contacts the programs emergency 800 number. Callers receive help on how to search the area, contact police, and report the person missing. The program will also create and distribute notices in areas where the missing person may have traveled. Finally, Safe Return will help the family prevent future wandering when the person is returned home.

Respite care

Caregiver respite should be made a priority and addressed at each visit. Gentle reminders to marshal the resources available within extended family or social circles should be given. At times, a more formal respite arrangement may be needed. Surprisingly, caregivers often resist suggestions for respite. They may feel guilty about their negative feelings toward caregiving, and they may also have difficulty entrusting their loved one to someone else. Unfortunately, it often takes a crisis to occur before caregivers use respite services [23].

Respite services are available in a number of forms. Adult day-care services and companion or home-care services allow the caregiver a few hours to address their own needs. Other respite options include assisted living communities and board-and-care homes. In extreme situations, admission of the patient to a nursing home or hospital might be considered.

Finding the right respite plan for the family takes time and will have to be modified as the disease progresses. Informal respite can be increasingly difficult to obtain as the patient's cognition and function decline, and the family will have to pay for respite services. Respite expenses may have financial benefits in the long term however, because respite services may delay long-term care placement [20].

Long-term care placement

As the caregiving burden increases, long-term care placement may become necessary to safeguard patients and meet their custodial care needs. The decision to place a loved one in a nursing facility is emotion laden, and conversations regarding it are difficult. Institutionalization may be considered culturally or morally unacceptable to some patients. Regardless, the possibility of long-term care placement needs to be addressed early because of its profound effect on the family's finances.

Long-term residential facilities that offer specialized care for dementia patients are commonplace. These facilities provide a safe environment for the patient, minimize disruptive behaviors, and offer structured activities. Currently, there are no standards that define long-term dementia care. Families need to take the time investigate the quality of care provided by the facility by meeting with the administrators, staff, residents, and their family members

Once the patient is admitted to a long-term care facility, their medical care is likely to be directed by a staff physician. On occasion, a patient or caregiver dissatisfied with the care received in the long-term care facility will contact the primary care physician. In this case, a referral to an ombudsman may help. Ombudsman programs are federally mandated to manage conflict between long-term care facilities and their residents. Information regarding ombudsman programs should be given to families at the time nursing home placement is considered. Contact information for ombudsman's offices is available through county health departments, the local office on aging, and the Alzheimer's Association.

Hospice care–help at the end of life

Hospice care is available in some communities for patients with end-stage dementia. These patients must carry a terminal prognosis of 6 months or less. Medicare criteria for this prognosis includes a Karnofsky Performance Status or Palliative Performance Score $\leq$ 70%, dependence on assistance for two or more ADLs, stage 7 or beyond on the Functional Assessment Staging (FAST) Scale, and any one of the following in the past 12 months: aspiration pneumonia, pylenopheritis or upper urinary tract infection, septicemia, decubitus ulcers, fever that recurs after antibiotic, inability to maintain sufficient fluid and calorie intake with a 10% weight loss in the previous 6 months, or serum albuin < 2.5 g/dL.

Hospice philosophy focuses care on patient comfort and family support and endeavors to maintain the patient's dignity while allowing for the natural progression of the disease. Hospice care should be considered when a patient no longer benefits from the services provided by routine dementia care programs. It is available in several settings including homes, long-term care facilities, and specialized inpatient hospice centers.

Summary

Dementia is a complicated disease state. It affects the very essence of who a person is and how he or she interacts with the physical and social environments. Given the complexity of the illness and the frequent need for care to be delivered through proxies (ie, the caregivers), disciplines beyond traditional medicine can provide useful resources for patients and families. Families expect that physicians will know about these resources and the ways they may help. Finally referral to outside resources can reduce the emotional, time, and financial burdens of dementia care for the physician. Sharing the load with other disciplines allows each to focus its own background, experience, and expertise on the needs of the patient and facilitate optimal long-term outcomes.

Acknowledgments

The authors wish to thank Stephen J. Modafferi, JD, for his gracious assistance in developing the content for this article.

References

[1] Pfeffer R, Kurosaki T, Harrah T, et al. Measurement of functional activities of older adults in the community. J Gerontol 1982;37:323–9.
[2] National Chronic Care Consortium and the Alzheimer's Association. Tools for the assessment and treatment of dementia in managed care settings. Bloomington (MN): National Chronic Care Consortium; 1999.
[3] Eisdorfer C, Rabins PV, Reisberg B. Alzheimer's disease: caring for the caregiver. Patient Care: The Practical Journal for Primary Care Physicians 1991;25:49–59.
[4] Corcoran MA. Gender differences in dementia management plans of spousal caregivers: implications for occupational therapy. Am J Occup Therap 1992;46:1006–11.
[5] Montgomery RV, Deawyler MM. Women and men in the caregiving role. Generations 1990; 14:34–8.
[6] Kiecolt-Glaser JK, Glaser R, Shuttleworth EC. Chronic stress and immunity in family caregivers of Alzheimer's disease victims. Psychosom Med 1987;49:523–35.
[7] Gallager D, Rose J, Rivera P, et al. Prevalence of depression in family caregivers. Gerontologist 1989;29:449–56.
[8] Bass DM, McClendon MJ, Deimling GT, Mukherjee S. The influence of diagnosed mental impairment on family caregiver strain. J Gerontol 1994;49:S146–55.
[9] Verhey FR, Jolles J, Ponds RW, et al. Diagnosing dementia: a comparison between a monodisciplinary and a multidisciplinary approach. J Neuropsychiatry Clin Neurosci 1993;5:78–85.
[10] Guttman M, Stober J. The social worker: an important part of the Parkinson multidisciplinary team. Parkinson Report 1999;10:9–11.
[11] Foley J. The experience of being demented. In: Binstock RH, Post SG, Whitehouse PJ, editors. Dementia and aging: ethics, values and policy choices. Baltimore (MD): The Johns Hopkins University Press; 1992. p. 30–43.
[12] Lachs M, Williams C, O'Brien S, et al. Risk factors for reported elder abuse and neglect: a nine-year observational cohort study. Gerontologist 1997;37:469–74.
[13] Reynolds JP. Working around dementia. PT Magazine 1995;3:64–79.
[14] Rouse J, Gilster S. An improved method of documenting and evaluating nutritional intake of persons with Alzheimer's disease. J Nutr Elder 1994;14:45–55.
[15] Matteson AM, McConnell ES. Gerontological nursing: concepts and practice. Philadelphia: WB Saunders; 1988.
[16] Carpenito LJ. Nursing diagnosis: application to clinical practice. 6th edition. Philadelphia: JB Lippincott Co.; 1995.

[17] Christopher A. Initial legal considerations of Alzheimer patients: process and form. Am J Alzheimers Dis 1996;11:25–8.
[18] Reckman MS, Seiler LH. Mental competency and planning for disability. Caring 1991;10:53–6.
[19] Hadjistavropoulos T, Taylor S, Tuokko H, Beattie B. Neuropsychological deficits, caregivers' perception of deficits and caregiver burden. J Am Geriatr Soc 1994;42:308–14.
[20] Dunkin J, Anderson-Hanley C. Dementia caregiver burden: a review of the literature and guidelines for assessment and intervention. Neurology 1998;51(Suppl 1):S53–60.
[21] Costa PT, Williams TF, Somerfield M, et al. Early identification of Alzheimer's disease and related dementias. Clinical practice guideline, quick reference guide for clinicians. No. 19. Rockville (MD): US Department of Health and Human Services, Public Health Service. Agency for Healthcare Policy and Research, AHCPR Publication No. 97–0703; November 1996.
[22] Katz S, Ford AB, Moskowitz RW, et al. Studies of illness in the aged. The index of ADL: a standardized measure of biological and psychosocial function. JAMA 1963;185:914–9.
[23] Adler G, Ott L, Jelinski M, et al. Institutional respite care: benefits and risks for dementia patients and caregivers. Int Psychogeriatr 1993;5:67–77.

ELSEVIER
SAUNDERS

Clin Geriatr Med 20 (2004) 141–152

CLINICS IN
GERIATRIC
MEDICINE

On the horizon: pathways for drug development in Alzheimer's disease

Ann Marie Hake, MD*, Martin R. Farlow, MD

Department of Neurology, Indiana University School of Medicine, 541 Clinical Drive, Suite 299, Indianapolis, IN 46202, USA

Alzheimer's disease (AD) is a progressive neurodegenerative disease that impairs memory, cognition, activities of daily living, and behavior. With the increase in the older population, the number of Alzheimer's sufferers will nearly triple by the middle of this century [1] unless treatments are found that can prevent or substantially delay the course of the disease. Pathologically, AD is characterized by the presence of amyloid plaques, neurofibrillary tangles (NFTs), decreased synaptic density, and neuronal loss. Neuronal loss is further hastened by inflammatory processes, free radical oxidation, and excitotoxicity. At a neurochemical level, deficits of cholinergic transmission are seen as neuronal loss occurs in the septal and basal forebrain nuclei, which project to the hippocampus and entorhinal cortex. Deficits of other neurotransmitter systems, such as serotonin and norepinephrine, also occur.

Current AD therapy is targeted at treating the symptoms of AD, mainly by working on the biochemical imbalances that are present. The mainstay of AD treatment for the past 10 years has been cholinesterase inhibition. Four agents are currently available for use in the United States: tacrine (Cognex, Parke-Davis, Morris Plains, New Jersey), donepezil (Aricept, Pfizer, New York, New York), rivastigmine (Exelon, Novartis, East Hanover, New Jersey), and galantamine (Reminyl, Janssen, Titusville, New Jersey). All four have been shown to produce modest but temporary improvements in cognition, global functioning, activities of daily living, and behavior. Their common mode of action is to increase the available amount of synaptic acetylcholine (ACh) through inhibition of the cholinesterases that hydrolyze ACh. Some recent reports have suggested that cholinesterase inhibitors may have slight disease-delaying effects [2,3]; however, more definitive therapies are needed. The goal of current research is to find disease-modifying treatments for AD by focusing on the underlying pathologic processes.

* Corresponding author.
E-mail address: ahake@iupui.edu (A.M. Hake).

doi:10.1016/S0749-0690(03)00073-9

Pathologic hallmarks of Alzheimer's disease

NFTs are intraneuronal aggregates of insoluble paired helical filaments. They are formed when tau protein becomes abnormally phosphorylated, which impairs its function of stabilizing the microtubules that compose the cytoskeleton. This causes dysfunction of axonal transport, which compromises cell structure, ultimately leading to neuronal death. NFTs tend to appear first in the entorhinal cortex and hippocampus, then gradually spread throughout the brain, and their distribution roughly correlates with the severity of the dementia.

Amyloid plaques form from extracellular deposits of amyloid β-protein (aβ). This protein is derived from a larger protein, the amyloid precursor protein (APP), which is synthesized within the neuron. As APP is extruded through the cell membrane, it is processed by various enzymes (secretases) to produce smaller proteins. α-Secretase is an enzyme that cleaves APP at a site outside of the cell membrane, producing soluble APP-α (sAPPα), which may have neuroprotective functions. The stub of the APP that is left protruding from the cell is hypothesized to have possible gene-regulating activities. However, an alternate processing pathway cleaves APP by β-secretase, which slices the protein at a site farther outside of the cell membrane, and γ-secretase, which snips APP within the cell membrane. The polypeptide fragment of APP that is between the cleavage sites of β- and γ-secretase is a poorly soluble, fibrillar 40–42 amino acid protein aβ, which has a propensity to aggregate in beta-pleated sheets in the extracellular space. aβ is neurotoxic; in addition, it promotes neuronal damage through oxidative damage, excitotoxicity, and promotion of inflammation.

Recent disappointments

Estrogen

Several epidemiologic studies reported a lower risk of AD in postmenopausal women taking estrogen replacement therapy [4–12], and several studies have shown a beneficial effect of estrogen on cognition in women [13–16]. However, two large randomized, double-blind, placebo-controlled studies of estrogen in women with AD showed no significant effect on cognition, ADLs, global functioning, or mood [17,18]. Recently, the Women's Health Initiative Study [19], a large, prospective randomized, double-blind, placebo-controlled study of hormone replacement therapy (HRT) in women, halted the combination therapy arm (conjugated equine estrogen and medroxyprogesterone) because of an increased risk of vascular events. Analysis also showed that twice as many of the emergent dementia cases occurred in the HRT arm as in the placebo arm (40 versus 21, respectively), and no difference was seen in the effect on mild cognitive impairment. However, the unopposed estrogen arm in women who have had hysterectomies has not shown these trends and is still ongoing, raising the possibility that the adverse effects of HRT may be attributable to medroxyprogesterone.

Anti-inflammatory therapy for Alzheimer's disease

The regions around β-amyloid plaques in patients with AD contain numerous activated microglial cells as well as elevated levels of acute phase reactants, complements, and inflammation-related cytokines such as interleukins 1 and 6 and tumor necrosis factor. Several large epidemiologic studies have suggested reductions of 30% to 70% in the incidence of AD in elderly patients who take nonsteroidal anti-inflammatory drugs (NSAIDs). The Baltimore Longitudinal Study, which prospectively identified medication use in longitudinally followed elderly patients, showed significant reductions in risk of AD for NSAID-taking patients; sub-analyses of this study suggested that risk of AD was even less for patients taking NSAIDs for 2 years or longer [20]. In most of these studies the average dosage was surprisingly low, equivalent to ibuprofen 200 mg twice a day. However, double-blind placebo-controlled trials with this class of drugs in patients with AD have been rare due to potential for significant risk of serious adverse events, such as renal failure, liver failure, and gastrointestinal toxicity including significant hemorrhage. Recently the development and availability of NSAIDs selective for cyclooxygenase-2 (COX-2), which were reported to have less gastrointestinal toxicity, have motivated large double-blind, placebo-controlled trials of both celecoxib and rofecoxib in patients with mild to moderate AD. Neither of the studies revealed significant benefits in delaying progression of AD [21]. The rofecoxib trial also had a naproxen arm. Patients on naproxen in this 1-year study also attained no benefits as compared with placebo, and greater numbers of significant hemorrhage occurred in both the rofecoxib and naproxen groups compared with placebo. Along with a previous large double-blind, placebo-controlled trial of prednisone in AD that was negative, these data have substantially dampened enthusiasm for anti-inflammatory approaches for treating AD [22]. However, NSAIDs may still be effective for primary prevention of AD. A very large double-blind trial of ibuprofen used for this purpose is in progress. It is possible that the older NSAIDs may prevent onset or delay progression of AD by mechanisms that are unrelated to COX-1 or -2 inhibition. It has recently been demonstrated that NSAIDs can reduce brain aβ levels, amyloid plaque burden, and microglial activation in an animal model of AD [23]. NSAIDs have also been shown to act as γ-secretase inhibitors [24–26]. However, on the basis of currently available clinical trial data, the evidence is equivocal or does not support the use of these drugs in AD.

Therapeutic targets in Alzheimer's disease

Glutamate

The most recently approved treatment for AD has focused on reducing impaired signal transmission and neuronal excitotoxicity via actions in the glutamatergic system. Glutamate is the major excitatory neurotransmitter in the brain.

In neurodegenerative conditions, including AD, mild chronic malfunction may lead to increased release of glutamate from both glia and neurons. This may produce an increase in the baseline calcium influx, which not only decreases the signal-to-noise ratio in neurotransmission but is also believed to produce long-term excitotoxicity and early cell death. This effect may be increased by the presence of aβ; in turn, excitotoxicity increases aβ levels, leading to an increasing spiral of neuronal death. Memantine, which was recently approved in the United States, is a noncompetitive antagonist of the N-methyl-D-aspartate (NMDA) subtype of glutamate receptors. It is thought to exert its effect by decreasing the excessive calcium influx at rest that occurs with glutamatergic dysfunction; however, it is easily displaced by glutamate so that it does not interfere with neurotransmission. Although it has not been shown to have disease-modifying effects, chronic administration could help preserve neuronal function by lessening excitotoxicity. Other NMDA antagonists are also being investigated as potential treatments for AD. In addition, earlier-phase studies of modulators of alpha-amino-3-hydroxy-5-methylisoxazolepropionic acid (AMPA) glutamate receptors are underway.

Glycogen synthase kinase-3

Glycogen synthase kinase-3 (GSK-3) is an enzyme that is intimately involved with both tau phosphorylation and with cleavage of APP by γ-secretase. Inhibition of GSK-3 may slow the formation of both NFTs and amyloid plaques. Recent studies have shown that the addition of lithium, a GSK-3 inhibitor, to cultures of rat hippocampal neurons results in decreased levels of tau protein [27]. Other studies showed that lithium and another unrelated GSK-3 inhibitor, kenpaullone, reduced the production of aβ in cell cultures as well as in a transgenic mouse model for AD [28]. Research is underway to test these compounds for clinical use, as well as to identify other compounds that may inhibit GSK-3.

Reduction of aβ and amyloid plaques

aβ formation is thought to be extremely important in the development of AD, because all the currently known genetic mutations that cause AD have been demonstrated to lead to increased production of aβ. For this reason, aβ reduction is a major target for potential therapy or prevention of AD.

Cerebrospinal fluid shunting as a therapy for Alzheimer's disease

Cerebrospinal fluid (CSF) turns over approximately four times per day in normal adults. In the elderly this rate may be halved, and in patients with AD the rate of production and turnover is even further reduced [29]. CSF circulation has been suggested as a pathway for clearance of potentially noxious metabolites including aβ. CSF shunting to the peritoneal space may increase the rate of turnover of these metabolites and may be therapeutic in patients with AD [30]. An alternative hypothesis is that CSF drainage containing higher levels of aβ than normally found peripherally may stimulate an increased immune response and production of antibodies to aβ that may have therapeutic effects in patients with AD.

In a 1-year feasibility study of shunting in 29 patients with mild to moderate AD, clinical and neuropsychologic testing at endpoint suggested stabilization of disease progression [31]. Examination of CSF at 1 year compared with CSF from baseline in a subset of nine patients revealed decreased levels of soluble tau as well as aβ1-42, a finding that would be consistent with the observed beneficial clinical effect of stabilizing disease progression. Interestingly, aβ antibody levels were also increased in CSF at 1 year [32]. A large multicenter double-blind dummy-shunt controlled trial of CSF shunting as therapy in AD is underway.

Secretase modulators

One possible approach to preventing the development of amyloid plaques is to inhibit β- or γ-secretase, or to promote α-secretase, thereby favoring the nonamyloidogenic pathway of APP processing. Several pharmaceutical companies are testing these compounds, especially γ-secretase inhibitors still pending, but published results are pending.

β-Sheet breakers

Another approach to inhibiting the formation of senile plaques does not focus on preventing the formation of aβ, but attempts to interfere with its formation into the β-pleated amyloid sheets. These compounds are essentially "decoys" that bind with aβ as if they were themselves aβ, but they do not contribute to the β-pleated conformation. This could theoretically prevent amyloid plaques from developing. A number of companies have compounds in early testing.

Immunization

Antibodies to aβ or humoral immunity may play a role in the natural clearance of this class of proteins. The hypothesis is appealing as these antibodies to both the aβ 1-40 and 1-42 forms of the protein have been demonstrated to occur in humans, and humoral immunity is known to progressively weaken with aging as AD becomes increasingly prevalent [33,34]. Studies initially undertaken in a mouse model for AD (PDAPP mouse) with vaccination using the aβ1-42 in young mice were able to demonstrate prevention of amyloid plaque formation over several months. Vaccination was then performed in older mice at an age when amyloid plaques are already abundant, and this approach to selectively stimulating the animals' immune systems was able to cause regression of established plaques [35]. Similar results were obtained in this and other transgenic mouse models by administering antibodies to aβ to the animal, rather than aβ itself [36]. These approaches generated some skepticism because such antibodies were not thought to cross the blood–brain barrier to have access to the amyloid plaques. However, more recent studies have demonstrated that a percentage of these antibodies do cross the blood–brain barrier. It has also been found that these aβ antibodies bind peripheral aβ proteins in the plasma, creating a potential sink that may draw aβ proteins out of the brain and amyloid plaques [37].

Vaccination with aβ has been tested in human normal controls, and in at least two studies in patients with mild to moderate AD by the Elan Corporation (Dublin, Ireland). In the largest study, 372 subjects participated in a randomized controlled trial. The study was terminated prematurely when ~ 6% of subjects developed encephalitis [38]. Autopsy results in one such subject revealed perivascular inflammation and an intriguing decline or lack of amyloid plaques in several areas of the brain [39]. Follow-up of treated patients is being continued to assess for possible clinical benefits despite interruption of the protocol. Although this trial was halted, considerable interest and enthusiasm remain for this approach and for peripheral administration of aβ antibodies. Studies will likely resume when mechanisms underlying both the beneficial and adverse consequences of this approach are better understood.

aβ Clearance

Another approach is to enhance the processes by which aβ is cleared from the brain, thus preventing accumulation and possibly causing regression of established plaques. Recent studies have revealed aβ-degrading properties of the metalloproteinases neprilysin and insulysin (insulin-degrading enzyme), and other candidate enzymes such as endothelin-converting enzyme and angiotensin-converting enzyme are also being investigated [40–42]. Plaque-clearing strategies that target abnormal metal accumulation within plaques are also being explored. Accumulations of metals including copper, iron, and zinc have been noted in association with amyloid plaques and are thought to potentiate the neurotoxicity of aβ. Two studies of chelating agents have shown some promise in AD. A small 2-year randomized, double-blind, placebo-controlled trial of the intramuscular chelator desferrioxamine (DFO) showed that those not receiving DFO declined twice as quickly in ADLs as the DFO treatment group [43], and later postmortem analyses of subjects who had received DFO revealed decreased brain concentrations of zinc and iron [44]. Another chelating agent, clioquinol, has advantages over DFO in that it can be administered orally and crosses the blood–brain barrier. Studies in transgenic mice revealed decreases of 50% or more in the amount of aβ present in the brain. A small open label study of clioquinol and B12 in patients with AD showed slight improvement in a 21-day trial, and a double-blind phase II study has also reportedly shown favorable results [45].

Cholesterol

In vitro and epidemiologic studies have suggested a role for cholesterol in promoting and for cholesterol-lowering agents delaying progression of AD. The addition of cholesterol to APP-expressing cell cultures results in decreased production of sAPPα, while addition of HMG-CoA reductase inhibitors (statins) to neuronal cultures lowers levels of aβ both intra- and extracellularly. Similarly, diet-induced hypercholesterolemia in rabbits and in AD amyloidosis-transgenic mice is associated with higher levels of aβ in the brain, while treatment with a statin blocks the aβ accumulation [46,47]. A study treating guinea pigs with simvastatin for 3 weeks did not reduce cholesterol, but did reduce lathosterol (a cholesterol precursor) and aβ by ~ 50% [48].

Epidemiologic studies comparing plasma lipid levels with the risk for dementia have shown varying results. A review of computerized medical records in three United States hospitals revealed the prevalence of diagnosed AD in patients taking a statin was 60% to 73% lower than the entire patient population over a 2-year period [49], and a case-control study using the UK-based General Practice Research Database revealed a reduction of risk for dementia of ~ 70% [50]. However, two very large prospective randomized, double-blind, placebo-controlled vascular prevention studies that have looked at cognition have shown no difference in rate of cognitive decline between the two groups [51]. To date there have been few controlled studies of the effects of statins in humans with AD. One small 26-week randomized placebo-controlled study in normocholesterolemic individuals with AD showed that simvastatin lowered aβ1-40 in the CSF of individuals with mild AD, but this effect was not observed in more severely affected subjects [52]. A large randomized double-blind placebo-controlled study of simvastatin in mild to moderate AD is in progress.

Homocysteine lowering

Although elevated serum homocysteine can be a marker for vitamin B12 or folate deficiency, multiple studies have shown elevated homocysteine to be an independent risk factor for AD even in the absence of low B12 or folate levels [53–57]. In a recent study, after correcting for other risk factors, elevated homocysteine was associated with a 2.9-times greater risk for AD than risk in volunteers with lower levels of homocysteine [58]. The Framingham study revealed that elevated homocysteine doubled the risk of developing AD [59]. It is thought that homocysteine itself plays a role in the development of AD pathology, as opposed to being a marker for other processes. Studies in primary neuronal cultures show that homocysteine potentiates copper- and amyloid β-peptide-mediated toxicity [60]. It is therefore reasonable to suggest that lowering homocysteine levels by folic acid administration may help reduce the risk of or slow progression of AD.

An 8-week pilot study of folic acid, vitamin B12, and vitamin B6 in subjects with AD did show a significant reduction in plasma homocysteine levels, especially in individuals who were not taking a multiple vitamin [61]. Another study showed that cobalamin/folate supplementation improved cognition in individuals with mild dementia and elevated plasma homocysteine, while no effect was seen in those with normal homocysteine levels or more advanced dementia [62]. A large randomized, double-blind, placebo-controlled study with folic acid, B12, and B6 is currently underway in patients with AD.

Antioxidants

Several studies have shown that that increased intake of antioxidants, either in the diet or through supplements, may help counteract the oxidative damage that contributes to neuronal loss in AD [63–65]. In the most widely reported antioxidant study for AD, subjects with moderate stage AD were randomized to vitamin E 2000 IU daily, selegiline 10 mg daily, vitamin E plus selegiline, or placebo. All three treatment groups showed significant delay to the clinical endpoint (progression to severe stage dementia, loss of two of three basic activities of daily living, institutionalization, or death), with the greatest difference being seen in the vitamin E group compared with placebo, with a delay of 230 days and 25% less deterioration in ADLs. No effect was seen on cognition [66]. Another study of high-dose transdermal selegiline demonstrated no significant difference from placebo [67]. Two randomized placebo-controlled trials of the coenzyme Q10 metabolite idebenone showed benefit versus placebo in mild to moderate AD [68,69], but a more recent long-term study was halted because insufficient efficacy. A small randomized, placebo-controlled study of coenzyme Q10 in Parkinson's disease showed a decrease in functional disability in the treated groups compared with placebo [70], but no trials of coenzyme Q10 in AD have been published.

Ginkgo biloba

Ginkgo biloba has long been touted as a natural, over-the-counter medication to improve or preserve memory. In vitro, ginkgo appears to have antioxidant, antiapoptotic, and antiamyloid properties. A 52-week randomized, double-blind, placebo-controlled trial of ginkgo biloba extract 40 mg three times a day showed slight improvement in cognition and global functioning in the treated group, compared with worsening in the placebo group. Although the difference between the groups was statistically significant, the clinical difference was negligible (a difference of 1.3 points change from baseline on the ADAS-Cog) [71]. Another large randomized, double-blind, placebo-controlled study of high dose ginkgo biloba extract (240 mg daily) is not yet published, and a very large, NIH-sponsored 5-year randomized, double-blind, placebo-controlled study for the prevention of AD in subjects over 75 years old is underway [72].

Benzodiazepine receptor modulators

Benzodiazepine receptors are roughly divided into two subtypes: central and peripheral. The best known are the central benzodiazepine receptors, which are concentrated in the central nervous system (CNS), are stimulated by agents such as diazepam or clonazepam, enhance the activity of gamma-amino butyric acid (GABA) through interactions with GABA-A receptors, and have sedative, anxiolytic, anticonvulsant, and muscle relaxant properties. Agents that are inverse agonists of these receptors have been found to improve measures of attention in animal and early-phase human trials. The peripheral receptors, which are found throughout the body, do not interact with the GABA-ergic system. It has been shown in animal studies that peripheral benzodiazepine receptors increase in the CNS with brain ischemia or injury, and it is thought that they are associated with glial cells. Inhibition of peripheral-type benzodiazepine receptors could promote brain tissue recovery by inhibiting glial proliferation and cytokine production. [73].

Summary

Available treatments for AD target its symptoms but do not significantly alter its course. Although today's treatments are greatly improved, a successful disease-modifying treatment for AD is desperately needed in the face of its rising prevalence and the enormous burdens it places on individuals and society. Fortunately, many promising avenues exist for development of a definitive treatment for this devastating disease.

References

[1] Ernst RL, Hay JW. The US economic and social costs of Alzheimer disease revisited. Am J Public Health 1994;84:1261–4.

[2] Doody RS, Geldmacher DS, Gordon B, Perdomo CA, Pratt RD, for the Donepezil Study Group. Open-label, multicenter, phase 3 extension study of the safety and efficacy of donepezil in patients with Alzheimer disease. Arch Neurol 2001;58:427–33.

[3] Farlow M, Potkin S, Koumaras B, Veach J, Mirski D. Analysis of outcome in retrieved drop-out patients in a rivastigmine versus placebo, 26-week. Alzheimer's disease trial. Arch Neurol 2003;60:843–8.

[4] Henderson VW, Paganini-Hill A, Emanuel CK, et al. Estrogen replacement therapy in older women: comparison between Alzheimer disease cases and nondemented control groups. Arch Neuron 1994;51:896–900.

[5] Waring SC, Rocca WA, Petersen RC, O'Brien PC, Tangalos EG, Kokmen E. Postmenopausal estrogen replacement therapy and risk of AD: a population-based study. Neurology 1999; 52:965–70.

[6] Steffens DC, Norton MC, Plassman BL, et al. Enhanced cognitive performance with estrogen use in nondemented community-dwelling older women. J Am Geriatr Soc 1999;47:1171–5.

[7] Baldereschi M, DiCarlo A, Lepore V, et al. Estrogen-replacement therapy and Alzheimer disease in the Italian Longitudinal Study on Aging. Neurology 1998;50:996–1002.

[8] Tang MX, Jacobs D, Stern Y, et al. Effect of estrogen during menopause on risk and age at onset of Alzheimer disease. Lancet 1996;348:429–32.

[9] Jacobs DM, Tang MX, Stern Y, et al. Cognitive function in nondemented older women who took estrogen after menopause. Neurology 1998;50:368–73.

[10] Matthews K, Cauley J, Yaffe K, Zmuda JM. Estrogen replacement therapy and cognitive decline in older community women. J Am Geriatr Soc 1999;47:518–23.

[11] Kawas C, Resnick SM, Morrison A, et al. A prospective study of estrogen replacement therapy and the risk of developing Alzheimer disease: the Baltimore Longitudinal Study on Aging. Neurology 1997;48:1517–21.

[12] Brenner DE, Kukull WA, Stergachis A, et al. Postmenopausal estrogen replacement therapy and the risk of Alzheimer disease: a population-based case-control study. Am J Epidemiol 1994;140:262–7.
[13] Phillips S, Sherwin BB. Effects of estrogen on memory function in surgically menopausal women. Psychoneuroendocrinol 1992;17:485–95.
[14] Sherwin BB. Estrogen and/or androgen replacement therapy and cognitive functioning in surgically menopausal women. Psychoneuroendocrinol 1998;13:345–57.
[15] Kampen DL, Sherwin BB. Estrogen use and verbal memory in healthy postmenopausal women. Obstet Gynecol 1994;83:979–83.
[16] Maki PM, Rich JB, Rosenbaum RS. Implicit memory varies across the menstrual cycle: estrogen effects in young women. Neuropsychologia 2002;40:518–29.
[17] Henderson VW, Paganini-Hill A, Miller BL, et al. Estrogen for Alzheimer disease in women: randomized, double-blind, placebo-controlled trial. Neurology 2000;54:295–301.
[18] Mulnard RA, Cotman CW, Kawas C, et al. Estrogen replacement therapy for treatment of mild to moderate Alzheimer disease. JAMA 2000;283:1007–15.
[19] Shumaker SA, Legault C, Rapp SR, et al. Estrogen plus progestin and the incidence of dementia and mild cognitive impairment in postmenopausal women: the Women's Health Initiative Memory Study: a randomized controlled trial. JAMA 2003;289:2651–62.
[20] Stewart WF, Kawas C, Corrada M, Metter EJ. Risk of Alzheimer's disease and duration of NSAID use. Neurology 1997;48:626–32.
[21] Aisen PS, Schafer KA, Grundman M, et al. Alzheimer's Disease Cooperative Study. Effects of rofecoxib or naproxen vs placebo on Alzheimer disease progression: a randomized controlled trial. JAMA 2003;289:2819–26.
[22] Aisen P, Davis KL, Berg JD, et al. A randomized controlled trial of prednisone in Alzheimer's disease. Alzheimer's Disease Cooperative Study. Neurology 2000;54:588–93.
[23] Yan Q, Zhang J, Liu H, et al. Anti-inflammatory drug therapy alters beta-amyloid processing and deposition in an animal model of Alzheimer's disease. J Neurosci 2003;23:7504–9.
[24] Weggen S, Eriksen JL, Sagi SA, et al. Evidence that nonsteroidal anti-inflammatory drugs decrease amyloid beta42 production by direct modulation of gamma-secretase activity. J Biol Chem 2003;278:31831–7.
[25] Eriksen JL, Sagi SA, Smith TE, et al. NSAIDs and enantiomers of flurbiprofen target gamma-secretase and lower Abeta42 in vivo. J Clin Invest 2003;112:440–9.
[26] Takahashi Y, Hayashi I, Tominari Y, et al. Sulindac sulfide is a noncompetitive gamma -secretase inhibitor that preferentially reduces Abeta 42 generation. J Biol Chem 2003;278: 18664–70.
[27] Takahashi M, Yasutake K, Tomizawa K. Lithium inhibits neurite growth and tau protein kinase I/glycogen synthase kinase-3β-dependent phosphorylation of juvenile tau in cultured hippocampal neurons. J Neurochem 1999;73:2073–83.
[28] Phiel CJ, Wilson CA, Lee V, Klein PS. GSK-3α regulates production of Alzheimer's disease amyloid-β peptides. Nature 2003;423:435–9.
[29] Silverberg GD, Heit G, Huhn S, Jaffe RA, Chang SD, Bront-Stewart H, et al. The cerebrospinal fluid production rate is reduced in dementia of the Alzheimer's type. Neurology 2001;57: 1763–6.
[30] Rubenstein E. Relationship of senescence of cerebrospinal fluid circulatory system to dementias of the aged. Lancet 1998;351:283–5.
[31] Silverberg GD, Leventhal E, Sullivan EV, et al. Assessment of low flow CSF drainage as a treatment for Alzheimer disease. Neurology 2002;59:1139–45.
[32] Du Y, Lin S, McGuire D, Farlow MR. Cerebrospinal fluid drainage by shunt in Alzheimer's disease decreases Abeta levels. Neurology 2002;58(Suppl 3):A134.
[33] Du Y, Dodel R, Hampel H, et al. Reduced levels of amyloid beta-peptide antibody in Alzheimer disease. Neurology 2001;57:801–5.
[34] Hyman BT, Smith C, Buldyrev I, Whelan C, et al. Autoantiodies to amyloid-beta and Alzheimer's disease. Ann Neurol 2001;49:808–10.

[35] Schenk D, Barbour R, Dunn W, et al. Immunization with amyloid-beta attenuates Alzheimer disease-like pathology in PDAPP mouse. Nature 1999;400:173–7.
[36] Bard F, Cannon C, Barbour R, et al. Peripherally administered antibodies against amyloid beta-peptide enter the central nervous system and reduce pathology in a mouse model of Alzheimer's disease. Nat Med 2000;6:916–9.
[37] DeMattos RB, Bales KR, Cummins D, Dodel JC, Paul SM. Peripheral anti A beta antibody alters CNS and plasma A beta clearance and decreases brain A beta burden in a mouse model of Alzheimer's disease. Proc Natl Acad Sci USA 2001;98:8850–5.
[38] Senior K. Dosing in a phase II trial of Alzheimer's vaccine suspended. Lancet Neurol 2002; 1:3.
[39] Nicoll JAR, Wilkinson D, Holmes C, et al. Neuropathology of human Alzheimer disease after immunization with amyloid-β peptide: a case report. Nat Med 2003;9:448–52.
[40] Iwata N, Tsubuki S, Takaki Y, et al. Metabolic regulation of brain Abeta by neprilysin. Science 2001;292(5521):1550–2.
[41] Farris W, Mansourian S, Chang Y, et al. Insulin-degrading enzyme regulates the levels of insulin, amyloid beta-protein, and the beta-amyloid precursor protein intracellular domain in vivo. Proc Natl Acad Sci USA 2003;100(7):4162–7.
[42] Carson JA, Turner AJ. β-Amyloid catabolism: roles for neprilysin (NEP) and other metallopeptidases? J Neurochem 2002;81:1–8.
[43] Crapper McLachlan DR, Dalton AJ, Kruck TPA. Intramuscular desferrioxamine in patients with Alzheimer's disease. Lancet 1991;337:1304–8.
[44] Cuajungco MP, Faget KY, Huang X, et al. Metal chelation as a potential therapy for Alzheimer's disease. Ann NY Acad Sci 2000;920:292–304.
[45] Finefrock AE, Bush AI, Doraiswamy PM. Current status of metals as therapeutic targets in Alzheimer's disease. J Am Geriatr Soc 2003;51(8):1143–8.
[46] Sparks DL, Scheff SW, Hunsacker III JC, Liu H, Landers T, Gross DR. Induction of Alzheimer-like beta-amyloid immunoreactivity in the brains of rabbits with dietary cholesterol. Exp Neurol 1994;126:88–94.
[47] Refolo LM, Papolla MA, LaFrancois J, et al. A cholesterol-lowering drug reduces beta-amyloid pathology in a mouse model of Alzheimer's disease. Neurobiol Dis 2001;8:890–9.
[48] Fassbender K, Simons M, Bergmann C, et al. Simvastatin strongly reduces levels of Alzheimer's disease beta amyloid peptides Abeta 42 and Abeta 40 in vitro and in vivo. Proc Natl Acad Sci USA 2001;98:5856–61.
[49] Wolozin B, Kellman W, Ruosseau P, Celesia GG, Siegel G. Decreased prevalence of Alzheimer disease associated with 3-hydroxy-3-methyglutaryl coenzyme A reductase inhibitors. Arch Neurol 2000;57:1439–43.
[50] Jick H, Zornberg GL, Jick SS, Seshadri S, Drachman DA. Statins and the risk of dementia. Lancet 2002;356(9242):1627–31.
[51] Shepherd J, Blauw GJ, Murphy MB, et al. Prospective study of pravastatin in the elderly at risk. Pravastatin in elderly individuals at risk of vascular disease (PROSPER): a randomised controlled trial. Lancet 2002;360(9346):1623–30.
[52] Simons M, Schwarzler F, Lutjohann D, et al. Treatment with simvastatin in normocholesterolemic patients with Alzheimer's disease: a 26-week randomized, placebo-controlled, double-blind trial. Ann Neurol 2002;52(3):346–50.
[53] Nilsson K, Gustafson L, Faldt R, et al. Hyperhomocysteinaemia – a common finding in a psychogeriatric population. Eur J Clin Invest 1996;26:853–9.
[54] Joosten E, Lesaffre E, Riezler R, et al. Is metabolic evidence for vitamin B-12 and folate deficiency more frequent in elderly patients with Alzheimer's disease? J Gerontol A Biol Sci Med Sci 1997;52:M76–9.
[55] Clarke R, Smith AD, Jobst KA, et al. Folate, vitamin B12, and serum total homocysteine levels in confirmed Alzheimer disease. Arch Neurol 1998;55:1449–55.
[56] McCaddon A, Davies G, Hudson P, et al. Total serum homocysteine in senile dementia of the Alzheimer type. Int J Geriatr Psychiatry 1998;13:235–9.

[57] Lehmann M, Gottfries CG, Regland B. Identification of cognitive impairment in the elderly: homocysteine is an early marker. Dement Geriatr Cogn Disord 1999;10:12–20.
[58] McIlroy SP, Dynan KB, Lawson JT, Patterson CC, Passmore AP. Moderately elevated plasma homocysteine, methylenetetrahydrofolate reductase genotype, and risk for stroke, vascular dementia, and Alzheimer disease in Northern Ireland. Stroke 2002;33(10):2351–6.
[59] Seshadri S, Beiser A, Selhub J, et al. Plasma homocysteine as a risk factor for dementia and Alzheimer's disease. N Engl J Med 2002;346(7):476–83.
[60] White AR, Huang X, Jobling MF, et al. Homocysteine potentiates copper- and amyloid beta peptide-mediated toxicity in primary neuronal cultures: possible risk factors in the Alzheimer's-type neurodegenerative pathways. J Neurochem 2001;76(5):1509–20.
[61] Aisen PS, Egelko S, Andrews H, Diaz-Arrastia R, Weiner M, DeCarli C, et al. A pilot study of vitamins to lower plasma homocysteine levels in Alzheimer disease. Am J Geriatr Psychiatry 2003;11(2):246–9.
[62] Nilsson K, Gustafson L, Hultberg B. Improvement of cognitive functions after cobalamin/folate supplementation in elderly patients with dementia and elevated plasma homocysteine. Intl J Geriatr Psychiatry 2001;16(6):609–14.
[63] Varner AE, Brenner S, Morris MC, et al. Antioxidants and risk of Alzheimer disease. JAMA 2002;288:2265–6.
[64] Morris MC, Evans DA, Bienias JL, et al. Dietary intake of antioxidant nutrients and the risk of incident Alzheimer disease in a biracial community study. JAMA 2002;287:3230–7.
[65] Engelhart MJ, Geerlings MI, Ruitenberg A, et al. Dietary intake of antioxidants and risk of Alzheimer disease. JAMA 2002;287:3223–9.
[66] Sano M, Ernesto C, Thomas RG, et al. A controlled trial of selegiline, alpha-tocopherol, or both as treatment for Alzheimer's disease. The Alzheimer's Disease Cooperative Study. N Engl J Med 1997;336(17):1216–22.
[67] Farlow MR, Tariot P, Hochadel T, Hake AM, Schneider L. Disease stage severity at baseline influenced progression rate in a 48-week selegiline Alzheimer's disease treatment trial. Neurology 1999;52(Suppl 2):A172–3.
[68] Gutzmann H, Hadler D. Sustained efficacy and safety of idebenone in the treatment of Alzheimer's disease: update on a 2-year double-blind multicentre study. J Neural Transm Suppl 1998; 54:301–10.
[69] Weyer G, Babej-Dolle RM, Hadler D, Hofmann S, Herrmann WM. A controlled study of 2 doses of idebenone in the treatment of Alzheimer's disease. Neuropsychobiology 1997; 36(2):73–82.
[70] Shults CW, Oakes D, Kieburtz K, et al, and the Parkinson Study Group. Effects of coenzyme Q10 in early Parkinson disease: evidence of slowing of the functional decline. Arch Neurol 2002; 59:1541–50
[71] Le Bars PL, Kieser M, Itil KZ. A 26-week analysis of a double-blind, placebo-controlled trial of the ginkgo biloba extract EGb 761 in dementia. Dement Geriatr Cogn Disord 2000;11(4):230–7.
[72] Schneider LS. Potential noncholinergic strategies for Alzheimer's disease. Geriatrics 2003; 58(Suppl 1):4–8.
[73] Maubach K. GABA(A) receptor subtype selective cognition enhancers. Curr Drug Targets CNS Neurol Disord 2003;2(4):233–9.

ELSEVIER
SAUNDERS

Clin Geriatr Med 20 (2004) 153–157

CLINICS IN GERIATRIC MEDICINE

Index

Note: Page numbers of article titles are in **boldface** type.

A

0749-0690/04/$ – see front matter
doi:10.1016/S0749-0690(04)00012-6

P

R

S

T

V

W

Changing Your Address?

Make sure your subscription changes too! When you notify us of your new address, you can help make our job easier by including an exact copy of your Clinics label number with your old address (see illustration below.) This number identifies you to our computer system and will speed the processing of your address change. Please be sure this label number accompanies your old address and your corrected address—you can send an old Clinics label with your number on it or just copy it exactly and send it to the address listed below.

We appreciate your help in our attempt to give you continuous coverage. Thank you.

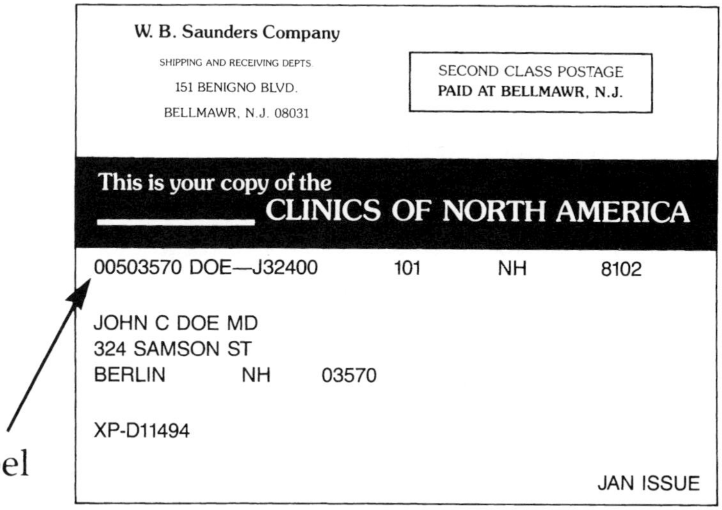

Your Clinics Label Number

Copy it exactly or send your label along with your address to:
W.B. Saunders Company, Customer Service
Orlando, FL 32887-4800
Call Toll Free 1-800-654-2452

Please allow four to six weeks for delivery of new subscriptions and for processing address changes.